HEALTHY LIVER, HAPPY LIFE

PROACTIVE STEPS AND LIVING TIPS FOR LIVER DISEASE.

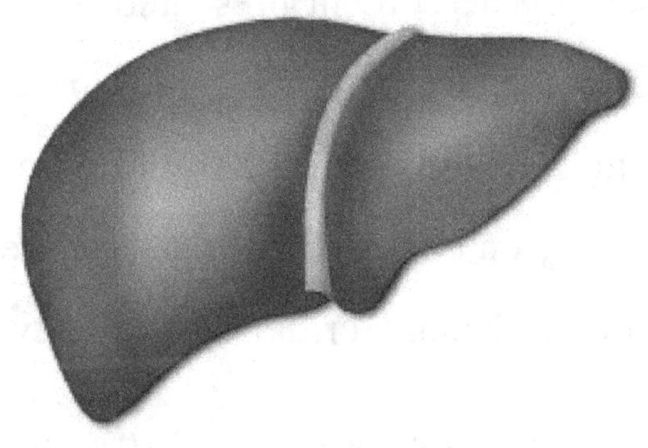

BY: DR. JADEN CLINTON

TABLE OF CONTENT

DISCLAIMER

Healthy Liver, Happy Life: Proactive Steps and Living Tips for Liver Disease is intended for informational purposes only and is not a substitute for professional medical advice, diagnosis, or treatment. Always seek the advice of your physician or other qualified healthcare provider with any questions you may have regarding a medical condition.

The information presented in this book is based on current research and best practices at the time of publication. However, medical knowledge and practices are constantly evolving. Readers are encouraged to consult with their healthcare professional for personalized guidance and to stay informed about the latest advancements in liver disease management.

The publisher and author do not assume any liability for damages or negative consequences arising from the application of the information contained in this book.

Please remember:

You are ultimately responsible for your health decisions.

Never disregard professional medical advice or delay in seeking it because of something you have read in this book.

INTRODUCTION

Imagine this: you wake up feeling energized, your mind sharp, and your body ready to conquer the day. This vibrant life, bursting with energy and well-being, isn't just a dream – it's the power you hold within your own body, specifically in a silent hero: your liver.

Think about it. Your liver, this unsung champion, tirelessly filters toxins, processes nutrients, and keeps your entire system running smoothly. It's the ultimate rock star, silently performing a symphony of essential functions behind the scenes. But just like any rock star, sometimes your liver needs a little support.

Here's the reality check: millions of people worldwide face liver issues, often due to factors like fatty liver, hepatitis, or even the occasional overindulgence. The good news? You're not powerless. This book is your backstage pass to unleashing the full potential of your liver and living a life that rocks!

Forget the passive approach. This isn't just about surviving with liver disease; it's about thriving. Packed with actionable tips, real-life examples, and the latest science, "Healthy Liver, Happy Life" is your roadmap to:

Decode Food Labels Like a Boss: Learn to navigate the grocery aisles with confidence, choosing foods that make your liver sing (and ditch the ones that don't). Remember Angela? She went from feeling sluggish and foggy to a fitness enthusiast by simply swapping sugary drinks for water and adding colorful veggies to her diet.

Move Your Body, Move Your Life Forward: Discover how exercise can become your liver's best friend, boosting its function and your overall well-being. John, a busy accountant, found his groove with brisk walks during lunch breaks, noticing a significant improvement in his energy levels.

Become an Advocate for Your Health: We'll equip you with the knowledge to communicate effectively with your doctor, understand your diagnosis, and make informed decisions about your treatment plan.

Build a Support System That Rocks: You're not alone on this journey. Learn how to build a network of support, from finding online communities to talking openly with loved ones. Remember Emily? After joining a support group, she discovered a wealth of tips and emotional support, completely changing her perspective on living with liver disease.

"Healthy Liver, Happy Life" isn't just a book; it's a call to action. It's about empowering you to take charge, make informed choices, and live a life that's vibrant, joyful, and full of energy. Let's face the music – your liver deserves a standing ovation. Let's give it one, together.

CHAPTER ONE

THE MIGHTY LIVER: YOUR BODY'S POWERHOUSE

1.1 UNVEILING THE LIVER: ITS ANATOMY AND AMAZING FUNCTIONS

Tucked away beneath your diaphragm, in the upper right quadrant of your abdomen, lies a remarkable organ: your liver. It might not be the most glamorous body part, but its importance is undeniable. Think of it as your body's unsung hero, silently working tirelessly in the background to keep you healthy and functioning at your best.

Built for Business: The Liver's Impressive Anatomy

Picture your liver as a reddish-brown factory, roughly the size of a football. It's divided into two main lobes – the right lobe being larger than the left – and further segmented into thousands of tiny hexagonal units called lobules. These lobules are the powerhouses of the liver, where most of the magic happens.

Blood vessels snake through the liver like a complex highway system. Unlike most organs that receive blood primarily from arteries, the liver gets its blood supply from two sources:

The portal vein: This large vein delivers nutrient-rich blood that has already passed through your intestines. This blood is loaded with the products of digestion – sugars, fats, proteins, and even some toxins absorbed from your food.

The hepatic artery: This artery supplies oxygen-rich blood from your heart, providing the necessary fuel for the liver's tireless work.

A Symphony of Functions: What Your Liver Does (and Why It Matters)

The liver is a true multitasker, juggling an impressive array of functions that keep your body running smoothly.

Here's a glimpse into some of its most crucial roles:

The Ultimate Detoxifier: Think of your liver as your body's internal filtration system. It processes and eliminates harmful substances like toxins, alcohol, and even some medications. These unwanted guests are either broken down into harmless components or packaged up for removal through your bile or urine.

The Master of Metabolism: Your liver plays a central role in converting the nutrients from your food into usable energy. It breaks down sugars and stores them as glycogen, a readily available fuel for your muscles and brain. It also processes fats, helping to regulate cholesterol levels and providing essential fatty acids for your body's functions.

Protein Powerhouse: The liver is a major producer of proteins, including those crucial for blood clotting, immunity, and transporting hormones and vitamins throughout your body.

Storage Champion: Your liver acts as a vital storage unit for essential nutrients like vitamins A, D, E, K, and B12. It also stores iron, which is necessary for carrying oxygen in your red blood cells.

Blood Flow Regulator: The liver plays a critical role in regulating blood flow throughout your body. It produces a protein called albumin, which helps maintain the balance of fluids in your bloodstream and prevents swelling.

Building Blocks for Life: The liver produces bile, a yellowish-green fluid that aids in digestion by breaking down fats in your small intestine.

Red Blood Cell Recycling Center: Worn-out red blood cells are broken down and recycled by the liver, with components like iron being salvaged for new cell production.

This is just a taste of the incredible work your liver performs every single day. It's a complex and fascinating organ, and understanding its functions gives you a deeper appreciation for its importance in maintaining your overall health and well-being.

1.2 The Liver's Symphony: How It Processes Everything You Consume

Your liver is a maestro, conducting a complex symphony within your body. Every bite you take sets off a cascade of events, with your liver playing the lead role in transforming food into the fuel and building blocks your body needs to thrive. Let's delve into this fascinating process:

The Arrival of Nutrients:

Remember that two-way traffic system we discussed earlier? The portal vein, carrying nutrient-rich blood from your intestines, delivers the first act of the performance. This blood is packed with the broken-down products of your meal – sugars (glucose), fats (triglycerides and fatty acids), amino acids (the building blocks of protein), and even some digestion byproducts.

The Detoxification Stage:

Think of this as the overture, where the liver starts filtering out unwanted guests. It identifies and neutralizes toxins, medications, and even some harmful bacteria from your food. These are either broken down into harmless components or packaged up for removal through bile or urine. Medications, for example, may be chemically altered by the liver to make them easier for your body to eliminate.

Sugar Blues and Sweet Solutions:

Glucose, the main sugar derived from carbohydrates, takes center stage next. The liver acts like a conductor, regulating blood sugar levels. It pulls out excess glucose from the bloodstream and stores it as glycogen, a readily available energy source for your muscles and brain. When your blood sugar dips, the liver releases stored glycogen back into the bloodstream, maintaining a steady flow of fuel for your body.

Fat Chance: Breaking Down Fats for Energy

Fats from your diet also enter the picture. The liver breaks down large fat molecules (triglycerides) into smaller components called fatty acids. These fatty acids can be used for immediate energy or sent off for storage in fat tissue around your body. The liver also plays a role in cholesterol management, producing good (HDL) cholesterol and helping to remove bad (LDL) cholesterol from your bloodstream.

Protein Power: From Food to Building Blocks

Amino acids, the building blocks of protein, also get their turn in the spotlight. The liver can convert some amino acids into energy, while others are used to build new proteins essential for various functions in your body. These proteins include enzymes that aid digestion, hormones that regulate processes, and antibodies that fight off infections.

The Importance of Bile: Aiding Digestion

The liver doesn't just process nutrients; it also produces a yellowish-green fluid called bile. Bile acts like a powerful detergent, breaking down fats in your small intestine into smaller droplets, making them easier for your digestive system to absorb.

Waste Not, Want Not: Recycling and Elimination

The final act of the symphony involves waste management. The liver breaks down old red blood cells and other cellular debris, extracting usable components like iron for new cell production. Waste products created during these processes are then packaged up and sent off for elimination through bile excretion into your intestines or via your urine.

A Delicate Balance: Maintaining Harmony Within

The liver's ability to perform this complex symphony flawlessly is vital for your overall health. When this intricate system is disrupted due to unhealthy eating, excessive alcohol consumption, or certain medications, the consequences can be far-reaching. The next chapter will explore some of the signs and symptoms that might indicate your liver's symphony is out of tune.

1.3 When the Music Stops: Recognizing Signs and Symptoms of Liver Disease

Your liver is a resilient organ, capable of performing its incredible tasks day in and day out. However, just like any overworked musician, it can become strained and struggle to maintain its rhythm. When this happens, the smooth symphony of processing can turn into a discordant tune, and signs and symptoms may emerge, acting as red flags that something is amiss.

Liver disease can progress silently, often with symptoms appearing only when the damage is significant. Here are some key signs and symptoms to be aware of that can serve as early warnings:

The Warning Signs

Fatigue and Weakness

Feeling unusually tired and lacking energy is a common symptom of liver problems. A malfunctioning liver might struggle to convert nutrients into usable energy, leaving you feeling drained. Additionally, the liver plays a role in producing proteins that help maintain muscle mass. When liver function is compromised, muscle breakdown can occur, further contributing to fatigue and weakness.

Loss of Appetite and Digestive Issues

A reduced appetite or feeling full even after eating a small amount can be a sign of liver trouble. This may be caused by a buildup of toxins in the bloodstream, which can interfere with your body's natural hunger cues. The liver also produces bile for digestion. If bile production is disrupted, it can lead to difficulty digesting fats, resulting in nausea, vomiting, and diarrhea.

Pain and Discomfort in the Upper Right Abdomen

A dull or aching pain in the upper right side of your abdomen, just below your rib cage, can indicate an enlarged liver. This discomfort occurs because the inflamed liver pushes against the surrounding organs and tissues.

Jaundice: A Yellowish Tint to Your Skin and Eyes

One of the most recognizable signs of liver disease is jaundice, characterized by a yellowish discoloration of the skin and the whites of the eyes. This yellowing occurs due to a buildup of bilirubin, a waste product normally processed by the liver. When the liver cannot efficiently eliminate bilirubin, it spills back into the bloodstream, causing the yellowing.

Dark Urine and Pale Stools

Changes in your urine and stool color can also indicate liver problems. Dark urine, often resembling the color of cola, can be a sign of increased bilirubin levels in the blood. Pale or clay-colored stools may occur due to a lack of bile pigments in the stool, which are normally produced by the liver.

Itchy Skin

Intense itching, particularly without a visible rash, can be a symptom of liver disease. This is thought to be caused by a buildup of bile salts in the bloodstream, which can irritate the skin.

Easy Bruising and Bleeding

The liver plays a vital role in producing proteins essential for blood clotting. When liver function is impaired, the production of these clotting factors may decrease, making you more susceptible to bruising and bleeding even with minor injuries.

Fluid Retention and Swelling

Fluid buildup in the abdomen (ascites) and legs (edema) can occur in advanced stages of liver disease. This happens because the damaged liver can no longer maintain the proper balance of fluids in the body.

Changes in Mental Function

In severe cases of liver disease, a buildup of toxins in the bloodstream can affect the brain, leading to confusion, disorientation, and even coma. This condition, known as hepatic encephalopathy, is a medical emergency and requires immediate attention.

Be Aware, But Don't Panic

Experiencing one or two of these symptoms doesn't necessarily mean you have liver disease. Many of these symptoms can be caused by other conditions. However, if you persistently experience any of these signs, especially if you have risk factors like heavy alcohol consumption or a family history of liver disease, it's crucial to consult your doctor. Early diagnosis and intervention are key to managing liver disease and preserving your overall health.

CHAPTER TWO

A CRASH COURSE IN LIVER DISEASES

2.1 THE COMMON CULPRITS: FATTY LIVER, HEPATITIS, AND CIRRHOSIS

Just like any complex system, your liver can face challenges. This chapter explores three common liver conditions—fatty liver disease, hepatitis, and cirrhosis—examining their causes, symptoms, and potential consequences.

Fatty Liver Disease: When Too Much Becomes a Problem

Fatty liver disease, as the name suggests, is a condition where excess fat accumulates in liver cells. Imagine a hardworking factory worker overloaded with materials.

There are two main types:

1. Nonalcoholic Fatty Liver Disease (NAFLD): The most common type, not directly caused by alcohol. Factors like obesity, insulin resistance (a precursor to diabetes), and certain genetic predispositions contribute to NAFLD.

2. Alcoholic Fatty Liver Disease (AFLD): Caused by excessive alcohol consumption. Alcohol is broken down by the liver, and over time, this process can lead to a buildup of fat within liver cells.

The early stages of fatty liver disease often go unnoticed, with no obvious symptoms. However, as the condition progresses, symptoms like fatigue, abdominal pain, and abnormal liver function tests may appear. The good news is that fatty liver disease, particularly NAFLD, can often be reversed or managed effectively through lifestyle changes like weight loss, adopting a healthy diet, and increasing physical activity.

Hepatitis: A Spectrum of Viral Infections

Hepatitis describes inflammation of the liver, often caused by viral infections. There are five main types of viral hepatitis: A, B, C, D, and E, each with unique

characteristics and transmission routes:

1. Hepatitis A: Highly contagious, usually transmitted through contaminated food or water. It often causes mild illness with symptoms like fatigue, jaundice, nausea, and vomiting. It typically resolves on its own and doesn't lead to chronic liver disease. A vaccine is available to prevent hepatitis A.

2. Hepatitis B: Transmitted through bodily fluids such as blood or semen. Early symptoms may be mild or absent, but chronic infection can lead to serious complications like cirrhosis and liver cancer. A vaccine is available to prevent hepatitis B.

3. Hepatitis C: A bloodborne virus causing both acute and chronic infection. While acute symptoms can be mild, chronic hepatitis C can lead to significant liver damage

over time. Effective antiviral medications can now cure hepatitis C in most cases.

4. Hepatitis D: Can only occur in individuals already infected with hepatitis B. It can worsen the course of hepatitis B infection.

5. Hepatitis E: Primarily transmitted through contaminated water and most common in developing countries. It typically causes a self-limited illness, although it can be severe in pregnant women.

Cirrhosis: When Scarring Takes Over

Cirrhosis is the end stage of various liver diseases, including fatty liver disease and hepatitis. Think of it as a beautiful landscape ravaged by multiple wildfires. In cirrhosis, the liver becomes severely damaged and scarred, hindering its ability to function properly. Scar tissue replaces healthy liver tissue, impairing blood flow and disrupting essential processes like detoxification, protein production, and bile production.

Symptoms of cirrhosis can vary depending on the severity of the condition. Common signs include fatigue, weakness, loss of appetite, jaundice, fluid buildup in the abdomen (ascites), and easy bruising and bleeding. Unfortunately, cirrhosis is not reversible, but treatment can focus on managing symptoms, slowing disease progression, and preventing complications like liver failure.

Understanding these common liver conditions empowers you to take charge of your health. The next chapter will delve deeper into less common culprits of liver disease, including autoimmune disorders and genetic factors.

2.2 Autoimmune Attackers: Understanding Autoimmune Liver Diseases

While fatty liver disease and viral hepatitis are the major players in liver conditions, other, less common issues can also disrupt the smooth functioning of this vital organ. This chapter explores autoimmune liver diseases, where the body's immune system mistakenly attacks healthy liver cells, causing inflammation and damage.

Friendly Fire: The Basics of Autoimmunity

Imagine your immune system as a highly trained army protecting you from invaders like bacteria and viruses. In autoimmune diseases, this army malfunctions, mistaking healthy tissues for foreign threats. This friendly fire can wreak havoc on various organs, including the liver.

The Main Player: Autoimmune Hepatitis

The most common autoimmune liver disease is autoimmune hepatitis (AIH). There are two main types:

1. Autoimmune Hepatitis Type 1: This form typically affects women of childbearing age more than men. The exact cause is unknown, though genetic predisposition and environmental factors are suspected.

2. Autoimmune Hepatitis Type 2: Less common and often associated with other autoimmune diseases like Sjögren's syndrome or primary biliary cholangitis.

Symptoms of AIH can vary in severity and may include fatigue, weakness, loss of appetite, nausea, jaundice, and abdominal pain. Sometimes, there are no noticeable symptoms until significant liver damage has occurred. Early diagnosis and treatment are crucial to prevent further damage and complications.

Other Autoimmune Liver Diseases: Not a One-Size-Fits-All Scenario

Autoimmune hepatitis isn't the only autoimmune condition targeting the liver. Here's a glimpse into some other, less common conditions:

Primary Biliary Cholangitis (PBC): This chronic autoimmune disease affects the bile ducts, small tubes that carry bile from the liver to the intestines. It primarily affects women and can lead to progressive damage to the bile ducts, eventually impacting liver function. Symptoms may include fatigue, itching, dry eyes, and right upper abdominal pain.

Primary Sclerosing Cholangitis (PSC): This autoimmune condition affects bile ducts inside and outside the liver. It is more common in men and often occurs with inflammatory bowel disease (ulcerative colitis or Crohn's disease). Symptoms can include fatigue, jaundice, itching, and abdominal pain.

Unveiling the Mystery: Causes of Autoimmune Liver Disease

The exact cause of autoimmune liver diseases remains unknown. However, several factors are believed to contribute:

Genetics: A genetic predisposition may increase susceptibility to developing an autoimmune liver disease.

Environmental Factors: Exposure to certain toxins, medications, or viruses may trigger an autoimmune response in some individuals.

Diagnosis and Treatment: Working with Your Doctor

Diagnosing autoimmune liver diseases can be challenging since symptoms overlap with other conditions. Your doctor will likely use a combination of blood tests, imaging tests like ultrasound or liver biopsy, and possibly autoimmune antibody tests to diagnose the condition.

Treatment typically involves medications aimed at suppressing the immune system and reducing inflammation. In some cases, medications are combined with lifestyle changes, such as maintaining a healthy weight and avoiding alcohol and tobacco. The specific treatment plan will depend on the type and severity of the disease.

Living with Autoimmune Liver Disease: Taking Control

While there is no cure for autoimmune liver diseases, early diagnosis and proper management can significantly improve your quality of life. Following your doctor's treatment plan, maintaining a healthy lifestyle, and staying informed about your condition are crucial for managing these chronic conditions.

2.3 Genetic Blues: How Genes Play a Role in Liver Health

Virtualize our bodies as beautifully complex creations, woven together by the delicate strands of our DNA. Just like our daily habits shape our health, our genes also have a say in how resilient our liver is to diseases. By understanding genetics, we can be one step ahead in taking care of our liver.

Our Genetic Blueprint and Liver Health

Every cell in our body carries a full set of life's blueprints—our DNA. These blueprints, found in our genes, determine everything from the color of our eyes to our risk for certain illnesses. Some genes specifically affect how our liver works, how it processes what we eat, and how it cleans out toxins.

When Genes Vary: The Impact on Our Liver

Genes aren't one-size-fits-all; they come in different versions. These variations, known as single nucleotide polymorphisms (SNPs), can change how a gene operates. Some SNPs might make you more likely to get liver diseases, while others could actually protect you.

The Iron Overload of Hereditary Hemochromatosis

A well-known genetic liver issue is hereditary hemochromatosis. It happens because of changes in the genes that manage iron. Too much iron gets stored in the liver and other organs, which can lead to serious damage. Catching this early and starting treatment, like removing excess iron, can stop worse problems from happening.

Alpha-1 Antitrypsin Deficiency: When Proteins Go Awry

Alpha-1 antitrypsin deficiency is another genetic liver condition. It's caused by a glitch in the gene that makes alpha-1 antitrypsin, a protein that keeps our lungs safe from harm. If this protein isn't working right or there's not enough of it, it can build up in the liver and cause harm. Treatments focus on slowing down the disease's progress.

Wilson's Disease: The Trouble with Copper

Wilson's disease is when the body can't handle copper properly because of genetic errors. This leads to too much copper in the liver, brain, and other places. It can cause tiredness, liver issues, brain problems, and trouble moving. Finding this early and treating it for life is key to managing it.

Genetics Isn't Everything: Environment Matters Too

Remember, our genes don't set our fate in stone. Even if you're more likely to get liver disease because of your genes, things like your environment can trigger it. For instance, someone prone to hemochromatosis might only get it if they eat too much iron.

Understanding Your Risk: The Role of Genetic Testing

If liver diseases run in your family, genetic testing can help you know your risk. This knowledge lets you make smarter choices and keep a closer eye on your liver health with your doctor's help.

More Than Just Genes: Other Keys to Liver Health

Genes are just part of the story of liver health. What you eat, how much you move, whether you drink alcohol, and your exposure to toxins all play big roles. Choosing a healthy lifestyle, eating well, and drinking less are important, no matter your genes.

The great news is that our liver is incredibly tough. By being proactive, knowing your risks, and living healthily, you can support your liver in its crucial job of keeping you healthy. The next part will give you the tools to understand diagnoses and talk to your doctor effectively.

CHAPTER THREE

DIAGNOSIS AND COMMUNICATION: PARTNERING WITH YOUR DOCTOR

3.1 BLOOD TESTS AND BEYOND: UNDERSTANDING DIAGNOSTIC TOOLS

Your liver, often the unsung hero of your body's cast, works diligently out of the spotlight. Yet, when trouble brews within this vital organ, it sends out subtle distress signals. If you're worried about your liver's well-being, it's time to seek a doctor's expertise. Let's walk through the detective tools your physician might use to unravel the mystery of your liver's health and pinpoint the root cause.

Blood Tests: The First Clue

Blood tests are typically the go-to method for uncovering liver issues. These straightforward tests are like secret windows into your liver's operation, measuring various enzymes, proteins, and bilirubin levels in your bloodstream.

Liver Function Tests (LFTs): Decoding the Liver's Harmony

A thorough liver function test (LFT) includes several crucial measurements:

Liver enzymes: These proteins are the body's natural accelerators, hastening vital chemical reactions. When liver cells are damaged, these enzymes spill into your blood. High levels of enzymes such as ALT, AST, and ALP can signal liver inflammation or injury.

Bilirubin: This yellowish by-product is usually processed and expelled by the liver. High bilirubin levels, particularly alongside unusual enzyme readings, can wave a flag for liver distress.

Total protein and albumin: Your liver is a protein factory essential for many bodily functions. A dip in total protein or albumin can hint at liver malfunction.

Prothrombin time (PT): This test clocks your blood's clotting speed. Since clotting proteins are liver-made, odd PT results may suggest liver harm.

Beyond Basics: Targeted Blood Tests

Based on initial test results and your doctor's hunches, you might undergo additional blood tests to:

Spot specific viruses: These tests can detect markers for hepatitis B, C, and other liver-affecting viruses.

Check autoimmune indicators: Certain antibodies can signal autoimmune liver conditions.

Gauge iron levels: To screen for hemochromatosis, blood tests can track iron quantities.

Search for genetic clues: Sometimes, genetic tests are used to gauge your inherited liver disease risks.

A Closer Inspection: Imaging Tools

While blood tests give hints, your doctor might suggest imaging methods for a more defined view of your liver's state. Common imaging tools include:

Ultrasound: A harmless way to visualize your liver using sound waves, revealing its size, shape, and any oddities like cysts or tumors.

CT scan: This advanced X-ray technique produces detailed abdominal images, offering a sharper look at your liver and neighboring organs than an ultrasound.

MRI Scan: Using magnetic fields and radio waves, MRI scans generate precise liver images, aiding in distinguishing between liver disease types.

The Definitive Test: Liver Biopsy

In certain scenarios, a liver biopsy is the ultimate diagnostic step. A tiny liver tissue piece is collected and microscopically examined, providing a direct glimpse into the liver cells and the specific damage.

Making Sense of It All: Collaborating with Your Doctor

Navigating diagnostic tests can be daunting, but you're not in it alone. Your doctor will decode the test outcomes and clarify their significance for your health. Engage in dialogue, express your concerns, and partner with your physician to tailor a treatment strategy just for you.

3.2 Asking the Right Questions: Effective Communication with Your Doctor

Finding out you have a liver condition might throw you for a loop, but remember, being informed is your superpower. This chapter is your toolkit for mastering the art of conversation with your doctor, asking the smart questions, and stepping up as a key player in your health journey.

Teaming Up with Your Doctor

Your doctor is more than a healthcare provider; they're your ally in the quest for liver wellness. Clear, open communication is the secret sauce to getting top-notch care. Here's how to chat effectively:

Come Prepared: Scribble down your questions and worries before your check-up. List any odd symptoms and your health history, meds included. This prep work makes sure you use every minute of your appointment wisely.

Ask for Simplicity: If doctor-speak sounds like gibberish, ask for a plain-language version. Getting the gist of your diagnosis and treatment is key.

Speak Up: Got fears or doubts? Let them out. Your doctor's there to ease your mind and support you emotionally.

Listen Well: Tune in when your doctor talks diagnosis, treatment paths, and side effects.

Note It Down: Keep a record of the convo or ask for a printout. It's gold for remembering what was said.

Second Opinions Are Okay: If the treatment plan doesn't sit right with you, it's totally fine to get another doc's take.

Must-Ask Questions for Your Doctor:

- What's the name of my liver condition, and what sparked it?

- What's the stage and future outlook of my disease?

- What are my treatment choices, and what's up with their pros and cons?

- How should I tweak my lifestyle to handle my condition?

- How often do we need to check in on my liver?

- Any cutting-edge treatments or trials I should know about?

- How's this liver thing going to play out in the long run for my health?

Customize Your Questions

These starter questions are just the beginning. Depending on your unique situation, you might have more to ask, like:

- How will my condition affect my job or travel plans?

- What's the deal with pregnancy risks?

- Should I be getting any special shots because of my liver disease?

Remember, no question is a dumb question. The more clued in you are, the better you can navigate your healthcare choices.

It's Not Just Talk: The Silent Signals

Good talk isn't just about words. Eye contact, nods, and wearing your heart on your sleeve can make your doctor chats even better.

Be Your Own Health Hero

Stand up for yourself—you're the boss of your body. Partner with your doc, ask those crucial questions, and dive into your treatment plan. You've got this, and you're all set to manage your liver health and rock a happy life.

3.3 Building Your Healthcare Team: Specialists and Support Systems

Stepping into the world of liver health can seem like a daunting trek. But here's the heartening bit: you've got company on this path. This chapter is all about the folks and support networks that'll bolster you as you stride toward the best liver health possible.

Your Health Squad: Beyond Your Family Doc

Sure, your family doctor is your go-to for health stuff, and they're likely the first you'd chat with about any liver concerns. But sometimes, you might need to tag in a pro—a hepatologist. These are the wizards of the liver world, with extra training in all thing's liver, bile ducts, and pancreas. They're the ones with the deep dive knowledge on liver conditions and the know-how to handle them.

It Takes a Village: Meet the Rest of the Team

Your liver's needs might call for a huddle with other health experts. Here's who might join your team:

Gastroenterologist: They're all about the digestive system, which includes your liver. A hepatologist is like a super-specialized gastroenterologist, but sometimes you might see a regular one, too.

Nutritionist or Dietitian: These food gurus tailor a diet plan just for you, keeping your liver's needs in mind. They'll help you balance what you eat, manage your weight, and steer clear of foods that make your liver grumble.

Surgeon: If things get serious with your liver, surgery might be on the table. A skilled surgeon will walk you through what to expect, including the big talks about liver transplants.

Mental Health Pro: Battling a chronic liver issue is more than just a physical thing—it can mess with your headspace, too. A therapist or counselor can be your guide, helping you navigate the emotional waves that come with liver conditions.

Finding Your Tribe: The Strength of Support Groups

Going solo with liver disease can feel lonely and rough. That's where support groups shine. They're a bunch of folks who get what you're dealing with. You'll swap stories, cheer each other on, and pick up survival tips. These groups are out there, both in the digital world and around the corner.

Your Personal Cheerleaders: Family and Friends

Don't forget, your squad at home is key. Loop them in on what's up with your liver, and lean on them. That mix of heart-to-heart chats and their cheerleading can do wonders for your spirits.

So, keep this in mind: You've got a whole team rooting for you. With a solid crew of healthcare champs, the camaraderie of support groups, and the love from your personal fan club, you're well-equipped to navigate the journey to a healthy liver.

CHAPTER FOUR

EAT SMART, LIVE SMART: DIETARY STRATEGIES FOR LIVER HEALTH

4.1 DECODING FOOD LABELS: MAKING LIVER-FRIENDLY CHOICES

Your liver is like the unsung hero of your body, tirelessly purifying your system day in and day out. To keep this vital organ humming, it's essential to fuel it with the right nutrients. This chapter is your personal guide to understanding food labels and selecting choices that will keep your liver in top shape.

Decoding Food Labels: What to Look For

Don't be daunted by the barrage of figures on food packaging. Let's simplify the essentials you need to consider for a liver-friendly diet:

Portion Awareness: The serving size is more important than you think. It's the key to understanding the nutritional info, so keep an eye on it to avoid overindulging.

Caloric Balance: Calories aren't the enemy, but balance is key. Overdoing it can lead to weight gain, which is extra baggage your liver doesn't need.

Fats to Favor and Avoid: Steer clear of the bad fats—saturated and trans fats—and embrace the good ones like those in olive oil, avocados, and nuts, but remember, moderation is your friend.

Cholesterol Check: Keep an eye on cholesterol, especially in animal-based foods. opt for leaner proteins and dairy that's low in fat or fat-free.

Sodium Savvy: Too much salt can cause trouble, especially if you're managing liver issues. Aim for a diet low in sodium to keep things in check.

Carb Quality: Choose complex carbs found in whole grains, fruits, and veggies for their nutrients and energy. Simple carbs? Not so much. They can mess with your blood sugar and aren't great for your liver.

Fiber Focus: Fiber is your digestive system's pal. It also keeps your blood sugar steady. Whole grains and fruits with their skins are excellent sources.

Sugar Smarts: Watch out for added sugars—they're the sneaky culprits behind calorie overload and blood sugar chaos. Go for natural sweetness from fruits when you can.

Micro Matters: Vitamins and minerals are your liver's little helpers. Foods rich in vitamins A, C, E, and the B's, plus minerals like zinc and selenium, are what you're after.

Ingredients to Be Wary Of

Beyond the numbers, the list of ingredients can tell you a lot about what's liver-friendly and what's not:

Alcohol Alert: Your liver processes alcohol, so too much can be harmful. If you have liver concerns, it's best to limit or avoid it altogether. Artificial Sweetener Caution: Generally okay in moderation, but if you're unsure, talk to a health professional about how they might affect your liver. Preservative and Additive Watch: Processed foods often have these extras. They're not all bad, but less is more for your overall well-being.

Tasty Swaps for Liver Health

Eating for your liver doesn't mean giving up flavor. Here are some tasty alternatives:

- Swap fried foods for baked, grilled, or steamed delights.
- Choose omega-3-rich fish, lean poultry, or plant proteins over red meat.
- Pick whole grains instead of refined ones.
- Drink water, herbal teas, or black coffee instead of sugary beverages.
- Snack on fresh produce, nuts, or air-popped popcorn rather than processed munchies.

It's the little tweaks that can make a big impact. Embrace whole foods, limit the not-so-good stuff, and diversify with nutrient-dense choices for a scrumptious, liver-loving menu.

4.2 Nourishing Your Liver: Essential Nutrients and Foods to Prioritize

A garden flourishes when it's fed the right fertilizers, and similarly, your liver thrives when it receives the proper nutrients. This chapter will explore the crucial nutrients that are key to liver health and spotlight the foods that are abundant in these vital elements.

The Liver's Champions: Vital Nutrients for Peak Health

1. Proteins: Just as proteins are fundamental to life, they are equally essential for your liver to repair and renew itself. Focus on lean protein choices such as fish, poultry, legumes, lentils, and a controlled number of nuts to minimize unhealthy fats.

2. Fibers: Fibers ensure a smooth-running digestive system and help maintain blood sugar levels, easing the workload on your liver. Look to fruits (with their skin on), vegetables, and whole grains as prime sources of fiber.

3. Antioxidants: These potent compounds are the liver's defense against free radicals that can harm liver cells. Load up on antioxidant-packed fruits and veggies like berries, leafy greens, grapes, and carrots to support your liver.

4. B Vitamins: These vitamins are pivotal in many bodily functions, including metabolism and energy production. You'll find a healthy dose of B vitamins in whole grains, legumes, and leafy greens.

5. Choline: An indispensable nutrient, choline bolsters cell membranes and aids in managing fat metabolism within the liver. Eggs, liver (with moderation, as advised by your healthcare provider), and certain nuts and seeds are excellent choline sources.

6. Omega-3 Fatty Acids: Found in fatty fish such as salmon and tuna, these beneficial fats can diminish inflammation and enhance liver function.

Crafting a Liver-Friendly Menu: Foods to Embrace

With the essential nutrients in mind, let's consider the food groups to focus on for maintaining a healthy liver:

Fruits and Vegetables: Aim to fill half your plate with a colorful selection of fruits and vegetables. They're loaded with essential vitamins, minerals, antioxidants, and fiber, all crucial for liver wellness.

Whole Grains: Replace refined grains with whole options like brown rice, quinoa, whole-wheat bread, and oats. These grains offer lasting energy, fiber, and vital B vitamins.

Lean Protein: Incorporate lean proteins such as fish, poultry, beans, lentils, and nuts (in moderation) into your diet. Proteins are indispensable for cellular repair and regeneration within the liver.

Healthy Fats: Embrace healthy fats, including olive oil, avocados, nuts (in moderation), and fatty fish. These fats are important for nutrient absorption and cellular health.

Foods to Moderate or Exclude:

Excessive Sugars and Refined Carbs: Overindulgence in sugary beverages, processed snacks, and refined grains can lead to fatty liver disease. Choose natural sweetness from fruits (in moderation) instead.

Unhealthy Fats: Saturated and trans fats, often found in fried treats, red meats, and processed snacks, can overburden your liver. opt for healthier fat choices.

Alcohol: Processed by the liver, alcohol can cause significant damage when consumed excessively. Moderate your intake or avoid it altogether if you have liver concerns.

Salt: High sodium can cause fluid retention and additional health issues. Watch your salt consumption, particularly if you're managing liver conditions.

A Liver-Friendly Meal Plan Example:

Here's a sample meal plan demonstrating how to integrate these guidelines into your everyday meals:

- Breakfast: Oatmeal topped with berries and a modest amount of nuts

- Lunch: Grilled salmon accompanied by roasted veggies and brown rice
- Dinner: Lentil soup served with a whole-wheat roll and a fresh salad Snacks: A selection of fresh fruits, veggies with hummus, or a small portion of nuts

Keep in mind, this is merely an example. Your individual requirements might differ. Always consult a nutrition expert or your physician to tailor a meal plan that suits your tastes and health needs.

4.3 Moderation is Key: Managing Sugar, Salt, and Unhealthy Fats

Your liver is a master multitasker, juggling various functions to keep your body running smoothly. However, excessive amounts of certain substances can overload this vital organ. This chapter will focus on three key culprits – **sugar, salt, and unhealthy fats** – and explore strategies for managing them to promote optimal liver health.

The Sweet Downlow: Taming Added Sugars

Sugar provides readily available energy, but consuming excessive amounts can wreak havoc on your liver. Here's why:

Fatty Liver Disease: Fructose, a common form of added sugar, can be converted into fat by the liver. Over time, this can lead to a buildup of fat in the liver, a condition known as nonalcoholic fatty liver disease (NAFLD).

Insulin Resistance: High sugar intake can disrupt your body's ability to use insulin effectively, leading to insulin resistance. This can further contribute to fatty liver disease.

Taming the Sweet Tooth: Practical Tips

While eliminating all sugar from your diet is unrealistic, there are ways to manage your intake and protect your liver:

Read Food Labels: Be mindful of added sugars lurking in processed foods, beverages, and condiments. Pay attention to serving sizes and opt for products lower in added sugars.

Embrace Natural Sweeteners: Satisfy your sweet tooth with natural options like fruits (in moderation) or a sprinkle of honey or maple syrup. Remember, moderation is key.

Limit Sugary Drinks: Sugary sodas, juices, and energy drinks are loaded with added sugars. Swap them for water, unsweetened tea, or black coffee (in moderation).

Cook More at Home: This allows you to control the ingredients and limit added sugars in your meals.

The Salt Shaker Squeeze: Finding Balance with Sodium

Sodium is an essential electrolyte, but excessive intake can have negative consequences for your liver, especially if you have existing liver disease:

- Fluid Retention: High sodium intake can lead to fluid buildup, putting extra strain on your liver.
- High Blood Pressure: Sodium can contribute to high blood pressure, which can further strain your liver and other organs.

Taking Control of Your Salt Intake:

Here are some strategies to manage your sodium intake and protect your liver:

Read Food Labels: Pay attention to the sodium content listed on food labels. Look for low-sodium options whenever possible.

Go Easy on Processed Foods: Processed foods are often loaded with sodium. opt for fresh, whole foods whenever possible.

Season Wisely: Explore flavorful herbs and spices to add zest to your meals instead of relying solely on salt.

Limit Added Salt at the Table: Be mindful of how much salt you add to your food during cooking and at the table.

The Fat Factor: Choosing Wisely for Liver Health

Not all fats are created equal. While some fats are essential for good health, others can negatively impact your liver:

Unhealthy Fats: Saturated and trans fats found in fried foods, red meat, and processed foods can increase cholesterol levels and contribute to fatty liver disease.

Healthy Fats: Monounsaturated and polyunsaturated fats, found in olive oil, avocado, nuts (in moderation), and fatty fish, can actually benefit your liver health by reducing inflammation and improving cholesterol levels.

Making Smart Fat Choices:

Here are some tips for incorporating healthy fats into your diet while limiting unhealthy ones:

Limit Fried Foods: opt for baking, grilling, or steaming your food instead of frying.

Choose Lean Protein Sources: Select lean protein sources like fish, poultry, beans, and lentils, and trim excess fat from meat before cooking.

Embrace Plant-Based Fats: Include healthy fats from sources like olive oil, avocado, nuts (in moderation), and seeds in your diet.

Read Food Labels: Be mindful of hidden fats in processed foods. Look for products lower in saturated and trans fats.

Remember, Moderation is key. Even healthy fats should be consumed in reasonable amounts.

By following these tips and working with a registered dietitian or your doctor, you can develop a personalized plan to manage your sugar, salt, and unhealthy fat intake, promoting optimal liver health and overall well-being.

CHAPTER FIVE

EXERCISE: YOUR LIVER'S BEST FRIEND

5.1 FIND YOUR FIT: CHOOSING ACTIVITIES YOU ENJOY AND CAN MAINTAIN

Your liver is your body's powerhouse, and just like any engine, it thrives with regular movement. Exercise doesn't have to be about grueling gym sessions; it's about finding activities you enjoy and can incorporate into your daily routine. This chapter will explore the benefits of exercise for liver health and guide you towards finding your perfect fit.

The Body in Motion: Why Exercise Matters for Your Liver

Regular physical activity offers a multitude of benefits for your overall health, and your liver reaps significant rewards as well. Here's how:

Improved Blood Flow: Exercise increases blood flow throughout your body, including your liver. This enhanced circulation helps deliver oxygen and nutrients to liver cells and removes waste products.

Weight Management: Regular physical activity can help you maintain a healthy weight or lose excess fat. This is crucial for liver health, as excess weight can contribute to fatty liver disease.

Insulin Sensitivity: Exercise improves your body's ability to use insulin effectively, which can help prevent insulin resistance and its potential complications for your liver.

Reduced Inflammation: Physical activity has anti-inflammatory properties that can benefit your liver, especially if you have a condition like nonalcoholic steatohepatitis (NASH).

Overall Well-being: Exercise can boost your mood, energy levels, and sleep quality, all of which contribute to a healthier and happier you, which indirectly benefits your liver health.

Finding Activities You Love: Moving Beyond the Gym

The key to sticking with an exercise routine is finding activities you genuinely enjoy. Here are some ideas to get you started, regardless of your fitness level:

Walking: This simple yet effective activity is a fantastic way to get your body moving. Walk briskly outdoors, explore your neighborhood, or find a walking buddy for added motivation.

Swimming: This low-impact exercise is gentle on your joints and provides a full-body workout. Swimming is a refreshing option, especially during hot weather.

Cycling: Hit the pavement or join a spin class. Cycling is a fun way to get your heart rate up and enjoy the outdoors.

Dancing: Turn up the music and let loose! Dancing is a joyful way to get your body moving and burn calories. Find a style you enjoy, from Zumba to ballroom dancing.

Team Sports: Join a recreational sports team for a fun and social way to exercise. Basketball, volleyball, or soccer are great options.

Yoga or Pilates: These mind-body practices combine physical postures with breathwork to improve flexibility, strength, and balance. They can be a great way to de-stress and improve your overall well-being.

Making Exercise a Habit: Tips for Consistency

The best exercise routine is the one you can stick with in the long term. Here are some tips to make exercise a consistent part of your life:

Start Small and Gradually Increase Intensity and Duration: Don't try to do too much too soon. Begin with shorter workouts and gradually increase the duration and intensity as your fitness level improves.

Find an Exercise Buddy: Having a workout partner can provide motivation and accountability.

Schedule Your Workouts: Treat exercise like any other important appointment. Block out time in your calendar and stick to your schedule.

Make it Fun: Choose activities you enjoy, listen to upbeat music, or explore new outdoor locations to keep things interesting.

Track Your Progress: Seeing your improvement can be a great motivator. Use a fitness tracker or simply keep a log of your workouts.

Listen to Your Body: Don't push yourself too hard, especially if you're new to exercise. Take rest days when needed and pay attention to any pain signals.

Consistency is key. Even short bursts of activity throughout the day can benefit your health. Find what works for you, and gradually integrate physical activity into your daily routine for a healthier and happier you, with a liver that will thank you for it!

5.2 The Power of Movement: How Exercise Benefits Your Liver Function

Your liver is a tireless worker, processing nutrients, filtering toxins, and keeping your body running smoothly. Regular physical activity acts as a potent ally, supporting your liver function in several key ways. This chapter will delve into the scientific evidence behind how exercise benefits your liver health.

Boosting Blood Flow: Delivering Oxygen and Nutrients

Picture your liver as a bustling factory. For optimal function, it needs a steady supply of raw materials – oxygen and nutrients. Exercise acts like a pump, increasing blood flow throughout your body, including your liver. This enhanced circulation delivers the essential ingredients your liver cells need to perform their vital tasks efficiently.

Combating Weight Gain: Reducing the Fat Burden on Your Liver

Excess weight, particularly around the midsection, can contribute to a condition called nonalcoholic fatty liver disease (NAFLD). This occurs when excess fat accumulates in the liver, potentially leading to inflammation and scarring. The good news is that exercise can help you manage your weight and reduce this fat burden on your liver.

Improving Insulin Sensitivity: Keeping Blood Sugar Levels in Check

Insulin is a hormone that helps your body utilize glucose, a type of sugar, for energy. When you're physically active, your body becomes more sensitive to insulin, allowing it to work more effectively. This is crucial for maintaining healthy blood sugar levels and preventing insulin resistance, which can contribute to NAFLD.

pacify Inflammation: Soothing the Liver's Distress Signal

Chronic inflammation is a hallmark of many health problems, including liver diseases. The good news is that exercise has potent anti-inflammatory properties. Regular physical activity can help reduce inflammation throughout your body, including in your liver, promoting optimal function and cell health.

Beyond the Physical: Enhancing Overall Well-being

The benefits of exercise extend far beyond the physical realm. Regular physical activity can improve your mood, reduce stress, and boost your sleep quality. These improvements in your overall well-being can indirectly benefit your liver health. When you feel better mentally and emotionally, you're more likely to make healthy choices that support your liver, such as maintaining a balanced diet and managing stress effectively.

The Science Behind the Sweat: Studies Highlighting Exercise Benefits

Numerous scientific studies have established the positive impact of exercise on liver health. Here are a few key findings:

- A 2016 meta-analysis published in the journal "International Journal of Sports Medicine" found that exercise training significantly reduced liver fat content in individuals with NAFLD.

- A 2018 study published in the journal "Hepatology" showed that moderate-intensity exercise improved insulin sensitivity and reduced liver inflammation in people with NAFLD.

- A 2020 review article published in "World Journal of Gastroenterology" concluded that exercise is a cornerstone of managing NAFLD and reducing the risk of progression to more severe liver disease.

Remember: Consistency is key. Even small amounts of daily activity can significantly benefit your liver health. Find an exercise routine you enjoy and can stick with for the long term to reap the rewards of a healthier and happier you, with a liver that functions optimally.

5.3 Moving with Limitations: Tailoring Exercise for Different Liver Conditions

The power of exercise for liver health is undeniable. However, navigating the world of fitness can feel daunting, especially if you have a specific liver condition or limitations. This chapter will address these concerns and guide you towards finding safe and effective exercise routines tailored to your unique needs.

Finding Your Fit: Considerations for Different Liver Conditions

Nonalcoholic Fatty Liver Disease (NAFLD): If you have NAFLD, moderate-intensity exercise is generally safe and highly beneficial. Walking, swimming, cycling, and dancing are all excellent options. However, it's crucial to listen to your body and avoid strenuous activity that causes discomfort. Consult your doctor before starting any new exercise program.

Nonalcoholic Steatohepatitis (NASH): This more advanced form of NAFLD may require a modified exercise routine. Your doctor may recommend starting with low-impact activities like gentle walking or water aerobics and gradually increasing intensity as tolerated.

Cirrhosis: This condition can cause fatigue and limit your exercise capacity. Low-impact activities like chair yoga or gentle stretching can be beneficial. Always work with your doctor to create a safe and appropriate exercise plan.

Hepatitis: Depending on the type and severity of hepatitis, your doctor may recommend rest or specific exercise modifications. In some cases, moderate-intensity exercise can be beneficial, but it's crucial to listen to your body and avoid strenuous activity. Always consult your doctor before starting any new exercise program.

Safety First: Precautions to Consider

Listen to Your Body: Pay attention to how you feel during and after exercise. Stop if you experience any pain, dizziness, or shortness of breath.

Hydration is Key: Drink plenty of water before, during, and after exercise to stay hydrated, especially in hot weather.

Warm Up and Cool Down: Always begin your workout with a gentle warm-up to prepare your body for activity. Cool down with light stretching after your workout.

Clear Communication with Your Doctor: Discuss your exercise plans with your doctor. They can provide personalized guidance and ensure your exercise routine aligns with your specific condition and limitations.

Modified Movement: Alternative Activities for Different Needs

Even if traditional exercise seems daunting, there are still ways to incorporate movement into your daily routine:

Take the Stairs: Skip the elevator and opt for the stairs whenever possible.

Park Further Away: Challenge yourself by parking further away from your destination and adding a walk to your errands.

Active Chores: Turn everyday activities into mini-workouts. Turn up the music and dance while cleaning, or park farther away and walk to the grocery store.

Chair Exercises: If mobility is a challenge, consider chair exercises like seated leg lifts, arm raises, and gentle stretches.

Recall: Every bit of movement counts. Start with what you can comfortably manage and gradually increase the intensity and duration of your activity as your fitness level improves.

The Power of Support: Finding a Fitness Buddy or Joining a Group Exercise Class

Exercising with a friend or joining a group fitness class can add a layer of fun and motivation. Look for classes designed for beginners or those with specific limitations. The support and camaraderie can make exercise more enjoyable and help you stay on track.

CHAPTER SIX

THE WEIGHT OF THE MATTER: MANAGING WEIGHT FOR LIVER HEALTH

6.1 UNDERSTANDING THE CONNECTION: HOW EXCESS WEIGHT AFFECTS THE LIVER

Your liver is a dedicated multitasker, and maintaining a healthy weight is crucial for keeping it functioning optimally. This chapter will explore the connection between excess weight and liver health, explaining how it can impact your liver's ability to perform its vital tasks.

The Domino Effect: How Excess Weight Overburdens Your Liver

Think of your liver as a well-oiled machine. When you maintain a healthy weight, it operates efficiently, processing nutrients, filtering toxins, and producing essential proteins. However, excess weight disrupts this delicate balance, creating a domino effect that can lead to liver problems. Here's how:

1. Increased Fat Storage: Excess calories are stored as fat throughout your body, including within the liver cells. This buildup of fat, known as fatty liver disease (NAFLD), can impair liver function.

2. Insulin Resistance: Carrying excess weight can make your cells less responsive to insulin, a hormone that regulates blood sugar levels. This can lead to insulin resistance, further burdening your liver.

3. Inflammation on the Rise: Excess weight often triggers chronic low-grade inflammation throughout the body, including in the liver. This inflammation can damage liver cells and contribute to NAFLD progression.

4. Metabolic Overload: Your liver plays a central role in metabolism, the process of converting food into energy. Excess weight increases the metabolic workload on your liver, putting additional strain on its resources.

From NAFLD to More Serious Conditions: The Potential Consequences

NAFLD, the most common liver disease globally, is often a silent culprit in its early stages. However, if left unaddressed, it can progress to more serious conditions:

Nonalcoholic Steatohepatitis (NASH): This more advanced form of NAFLD involves inflammation and liver cell damage. NASH can further impair liver function and increase the risk of scarring (fibrosis).

Cirrhosis: In severe cases, ongoing inflammation and damage can lead to cirrhosis, where healthy liver tissue is replaced by scar tissue. This significantly reduces the liver's ability to function.

Liver Cancer: While less common, individuals with advanced NAFLD or NASH have a higher risk of developing liver cancer.

The Importance of Early Intervention: Preventing a Cascade of Issues

The good news is that the connection between weight and liver health is a two-way street. Losing weight, even a modest amount, can significantly improve your liver health and reduce the risk of complications:

Reduced Fat Storage: Losing weight helps decrease the fat stored in your liver, alleviating the burden on liver cells and promoting healthy function.

Improved Insulin Sensitivity: Weight loss can improve your body's response to insulin, taking the pressure off your liver to manage blood sugar levels.

Taming Inflammation: Losing weight can help reduce chronic inflammation throughout the body, including in the liver, promoting a healthier environment for liver cells.

Decreased Metabolic Stress: By reducing your body weight, you lessen the metabolic workload on your liver, allowing it to function more efficiently.

Remember: It's never too late to make changes. Even a modest weight loss of 5-10% can significantly improve your liver health and reduce the risk of future complications.

6.2 Setting Realistic Goals: Sustainable Weight Management Strategies

Shedding excess weight can significantly improve your liver health. However, navigating the world of weight loss can feel overwhelming. This chapter will guide you towards setting realistic goals and developing sustainable strategies for achieving and maintaining a healthy weight for a healthier you and a happier liver.

The Power of Perspective: Reframing Weight Loss as a Journey, Not a Destination

Think of weight management as a journey, not a race to a finish line. Focus on developing healthy habits you can maintain for the long term, rather than quick-fix diets that are often unsustainable. Here's why a long-term approach is key:

Sustainable Habits Lead to Lasting Change: Crash diets and extreme calorie restriction may lead to initial weight loss, but they're challenging to maintain. Focus on building healthy habits you can incorporate into your daily routine for long-term success.

Slow and Steady Wins the Race: Aim for gradual weight loss of 1-2 pounds per week. This pace is more likely to be sustainable and lead to lasting changes in your body composition and overall health.

Small Wins Add Up to Big Results: Celebrate your non-scale victories! Increased energy levels, improved sleep, and better fitting clothes are all signs you're on the right track.

Setting SMART Goals for Weight Management Success

SMART goals are Specific, Measurable, Attainable, Relevant, and Time-bound. Here's how to apply this framework to your weight loss journey:

Specific: Instead of a vague goal of "losing weight," aim for something specific, like "losing 10 pounds in 3 months."

Measurable: Track your progress by weighing yourself regularly or using a body composition scale. Monitor changes in clothing size or energy levels.

Attainable: Be realistic about what you can achieve. A goal of losing 50 pounds in a month is likely unsustainable. Set a goal that challenges you but is achievable within a reasonable timeframe.

Relevant: Your weight loss goal should align with your overall health goals. Consult your doctor or a registered dietitian to ensure your target weight is healthy for your body type and medical history.

Time-bound: Set a deadline for achieving your goal. This creates a sense of urgency and helps you stay motivated.

Developing Sustainable Strategies for Healthy Weight Loss

Here are some practical strategies to incorporate into your daily routine for sustainable weight management:

Focus on Whole Foods: Fill your plate with nutrient-rich whole foods like fruits, vegetables, whole grains, and lean protein sources. These foods are naturally filling and keep you feeling satisfied for longer.

Portion Control is Key: Use smaller plates, measure your portions, and avoid mindlessly snacking. Pay attention to hunger cues and stop eating when you're comfortably full.

Mindful Eating: Slow down and savor your food. Turn off distractions like TV or your phone while eating. This allows you to connect with your body's hunger and fullness signals and avoid overeating.

Stay Hydrated: Drinking plenty of water throughout the day helps with hunger control and can boost metabolism. Aim to drink eight glasses of water daily.

Move Your Body: Regular physical activity is crucial for weight management and overall health. Find activities you enjoy and incorporate them into your daily routine.

Find Your Support System: Having a friend, family member, or support group can be a game-changer. Share your goals with someone who can motivate and encourage you along the way.

There will be setbacks along the way. Don't let them derail your progress. View them as learning experiences and recommit to your goals.

6.3 Building a Support System: Finding Encouragement and Accountability

The road to achieving and maintaining a healthy weight can feel more manageable when you're not alone. This chapter will explore the importance of building a support system, a network of individuals who can offer encouragement, motivation, and accountability on your weight management journey.

The Power of Togetherness: Why Support Matters

Let's face it, navigating lifestyle changes can be challenging. Having a support system in place can make a world of difference. Here's how a support system can benefit your weight loss efforts:

Motivation and Encouragement: Life throws curveballs, and there will be days when sticking to your goals feels difficult. A support system can provide a much-needed pep talk and remind you of your "why" – the reasons you're committed to a healthier lifestyle.

Accountability: Knowing someone is invested in your success can be a powerful motivator. A support system can hold you accountable for your choices and help you get back on track if you experience setbacks.

Shared Experiences: Surrounding yourself with others who understand your struggles can be incredibly valuable. You can share tips, celebrate successes together, and learn from each other's experiences.

Emotional Support: Weight loss is often more than just physical; it can have emotional aspects as well. A supportive network can provide a safe space to express your frustrations and challenges, fostering a sense of understanding and community.

Building Your Support Squad: Identifying the Right People

So, who should be part of your weight loss support system? Here are some ideal candidates:

A Weight Loss Buddy: Find a friend or family member who shares your goals or is also working towards a healthier lifestyle. You can hold each other accountable, share recipes, and motivate each other to stay active.

A Registered Dietitian: A qualified RD can create a personalized weight loss plan tailored to your needs and preferences. They can offer guidance on healthy eating habits, portion control, and navigating dietary challenges.

A Therapist or Counselor: Sometimes, emotional roadblocks can hinder weight loss efforts. A therapist can help you identify and address underlying issues that may be impacting your progress.

Online Support Groups: The internet offers a wealth of online support groups for weight loss. Connecting with others on a similar journey can provide a sense of camaraderie and valuable insights.

Beyond the Scale: Expanding Your Support Network

Your support system doesn't have to be limited to weight loss specifically. Building a well-rounded support network that promotes overall well-being can indirectly benefit your weight management efforts:

Friends and Family: Confide in your close circle about your goals and challenges. Their support and understanding can create a positive and encouraging environment.

Stress Management Techniques: Chronic stress can contribute to weight gain. Explore stress management techniques like yoga, meditation, or spending time in nature. Having a support system can also help you manage stress in a healthy way.

Join a Fitness Class: Group fitness classes can provide a fun and social way to get active. The camaraderie and support from fellow participants can keep you motivated.

Building a supportive network takes time and effort. Don't be afraid to reach out to different people and find a combination that works best for you.

CHAPTER SEVEN

REST AND RELAXATION: THE IMPORTANCE OF SLEEP AND STRESS MANAGEMENT

7.1 PRIORITIZING SLEEP: CREATING A RESTFUL ROUTINE FOR LIVER RECOVERY

While you sleep, your body isn't just catching ZZ's. It's a time of restoration and renewal, and your liver is no exception. This chapter will explore the crucial role sleep plays in liver health and provide tips for creating a restful routine to optimize your liver's function.

The Night Shift: How Sleep Supports Your Liver's Detoxification Process

Imagine your liver as a tireless factory, working around the clock to process nutrients, filter toxins, and produce essential proteins. During sleep, this factory enters a particularly productive night shift. Here's how sleep benefits your liver's detoxification process:

Enhanced Blood Flow: As you drift off to sleep, blood flow to your digestive system decreases and redirects towards your liver. This increased blood flow allows your liver to more efficiently remove waste products and toxins that have accumulated throughout the day.

Cellular Repair and Regeneration: Sleep is essential for cellular repair throughout your body, including your liver. During sleep, your liver can focus on repairing damaged cells and regenerating healthy new ones, ensuring optimal function.

Protein Synthesis: While you sleep, your liver ramps up protein synthesis, the process of creating new proteins essential for various bodily functions. These proteins play a crucial role in detoxification and overall liver health.

Hormonal Balance: Sleep is vital for regulating hormones, including those involved in metabolism and blood sugar control. Disrupted sleep can lead to hormonal imbalances that can indirectly impact your liver health.

The Sleep Deprivation Detriment: How Lack of Sleep Strains Your Liver

Chronic sleep deprivation – consistently not getting enough quality sleep – can take a toll on your overall health, and your liver is no exception. Here's how insufficient sleep can harm your liver:

Impaired Detoxification: When you don't get enough sleep, blood flow to your liver is reduced, hindering its ability to effectively remove toxins and waste products.

Increased Inflammation: Sleep deprivation can trigger low-grade inflammation throughout the body, including in the liver. This chronic inflammation can damage liver cells and contribute to fatty liver disease.

Disrupted Metabolism: Lack of sleep can disrupt your body's natural metabolic processes, potentially leading to weight gain and further straining your liver.

Increased Risk of NAFLD: Studies have shown a link between chronic sleep deprivation and an increased risk of nonalcoholic fatty liver disease (NAFLD).

Creating a Sleep Sanctuary: Tips for a Restful Night's Sleep

Knowing the importance of sleep for liver health, the next step is creating a sleep routine that optimizes your nightly rest. Here are some tips:

Establish a Regular Sleep Schedule: Go to bed and wake up at consistent times each day, even on weekends. This helps regulate your body's natural sleep-wake cycle (circadian rhythm).

Craft a Relaxing Bedtime Routine: Wind down before bed with calming activities like taking a warm bath, reading a book, or practicing relaxation techniques like deep breathing or meditation.

Create a Sleep-Conducive Environment: Make sure your bedroom is dark, quiet, cool, and clutter-free. Invest in blackout curtains, earplugs, and a comfortable mattress and pillows.

Limit Screen Time Before Bed: The blue light emitted from electronic devices can disrupt sleep patterns. Avoid screen time for at least an hour before bedtime.

Regular Exercise: Regular physical activity can improve sleep quality. However, avoid strenuous workouts close to bedtime, as they can be stimulating.

Avoid Caffeine and Alcohol in the Evening: Caffeine and alcohol can interfere with sleep. Limit caffeine intake to the earlier part of the day and avoid alcohol close to bedtime.

Manage Stress: Chronic stress can significantly impact sleep quality. Find healthy ways to manage stress, such as yoga, meditation, or spending time in nature.

Developing a consistent sleep routine takes time and effort. Be patient with yourself and celebrate your progress. If you continue to experience sleep problems, consult your doctor to rule out any underlying medical conditions.

7.2 Taming the Stress Beast: Techniques for Relaxation and Emotional Wellbeing

Chronic stress can wreak havoc on your health, and your liver is no exception. This chapter will delve into the connection between stress and liver health, and equip you with practical techniques to manage stress and cultivate emotional well-being for a healthier you and a happier liver.

The Stress-Liver Connection: How Chronic Anxiety Impacts Your Liver Function

Stress is a natural human response to challenging situations. However, when stress becomes chronic, it can take a toll on your physical and mental health. Here's how chronic stress can negatively impact your liver:

Increased Inflammation: Stress triggers the release of hormones like cortisol, which can contribute to chronic inflammation throughout the body, including in the liver. This inflammation can damage liver cells and contribute to fatty liver disease.

Disrupted Blood Sugar Control: Stress can disrupt the release of hormones involved in blood sugar regulation, potentially leading to insulin resistance and further straining your liver.

Unhealthy Habits: Chronic stress can lead to unhealthy coping mechanisms like overeating or increased alcohol consumption, both of which can negatively impact your liver health.

Weakened Immune System: Stress can weaken your immune system, making you more susceptible to infections that can further burden your liver.

Beyond the Physical: The Emotional Toll on Your Liver

The impact of stress goes beyond physical health. Emotional distress, such as anxiety or depression, can also indirectly affect your liver health. When you're feeling overwhelmed, it can be challenging to maintain healthy habits and prioritize self-care, both of which are crucial for optimal liver function.

Taming the Stress Beast: Techniques for Relaxation and Emotional Wellbeing

The good news is that you have the power to manage stress and cultivate emotional well-being. Here are some practical techniques you can incorporate into your daily routine:

Mindfulness and Meditation: Mindfulness practices like meditation can help you become more aware of your thoughts and feelings, allowing you to manage stress in a healthy way. There are numerous guided meditations available online or through apps.

Deep Breathing Exercises: Taking slow, deep breaths can activate your body's relaxation response, calming your nervous system and reducing stress levels.

Yoga and Tai Chi: These mind-body practices combine physical postures with breathwork and meditation to promote relaxation and stress reduction.

Spending Time in Nature: Immersing yourself in nature has been shown to have a calming effect on the mind and body. Go for a walk in the park, hike in the woods, or simply sit outside and soak up the fresh air.

Creative Expression: Expressing yourself creatively through activities like writing, painting, or music can be a powerful stress reliever.

Connect with Loved Ones: Social support is crucial for emotional well-being. Spend time with loved ones who make you feel good and offer a sense of connection.

Seek Professional Help: If stress feels overwhelming and is impacting your daily life, don't hesitate to seek professional help from a therapist or counselor.

Stress management is a journey, not a destination. Experiment with different techniques and find what works best for you. Building a stress-management toolbox will equip you to navigate life's challenges in a healthy way, promoting both your emotional well-being and your liver health.

7.3 Saying No: Setting Boundaries and Managing Mental Health

We all face situations that can trigger stress and overwhelm. This chapter will explore the importance of setting boundaries and managing your mental health for optimal liver function. Learning to say "no" and prioritizing your well-being empowers you to create a calmer and healthier lifestyle, ultimately benefiting your liver health.

The Burden of Unchecked Stress: Why Saying "Yes" Too Often Can Harm Your Liver

Constantly saying "yes" to requests and neglecting your own needs can lead to chronic stress, as discussed in the previous chapter. Remember, chronic stress can trigger inflammation, disrupt blood sugar control, and contribute to unhealthy habits, all of which can negatively impact your liver health.

The Power of Boundaries: Protecting Your Time and Energy for Optimal Well-being

Setting boundaries is about establishing healthy limits in your personal and professional life. It's about saying "no" when you need to, protecting your time and energy for the things that matter most. Strong boundaries create a sense of control and reduce stress, promoting emotional well-being and supporting liver function.

How to Set Healthy Boundaries:

Identify Your Limits: Be clear about what you can and cannot realistically handle. Consider your time, energy levels, and priorities.

Communicate Clearly and Assertively: Learn to say "no" politely but firmly. Explain your reasons without feeling the need to apologize.

Practice Makes Progress: Setting boundaries can feel uncomfortable initially. Practice saying "no" in low-stakes situations to build confidence.

Respect Others' Boundaries: Just as you deserve boundaries, so do others. Be respectful of other people's time and limitations.

Prioritizing Mental Health: Addressing Anxiety and Depression for Liver Health

Mental health conditions like anxiety and depression can significantly impact your overall health, including your liver function. Chronic stress associated with these conditions can take a toll on your liver.

Taking Care of Your Mental Wellbeing:

Seek Professional Help: If you suspect you may be struggling with anxiety or depression, don't hesitate to seek professional help from a therapist or counselor.

Develop Healthy Coping Mechanisms: Find healthy ways to manage stress and difficult emotions. This could include mindfulness practices, exercise, spending time in nature, or creative expression.

Build a Support System: Surround yourself with supportive people who understand and care about you.

Talking to loved ones about your mental health can be incredibly helpful.

Practice Self-Care: Make time for activities that bring you joy and relaxation. Prioritize good sleep, healthy eating, and regular exercise.

Taking care of your mental health is just as important as taking care of your physical health. By managing stress, setting boundaries, and addressing mental health challenges, you're creating a foundation for a healthier and happier you, and ultimately, a healthier liver.

CHAPTER EIGHT

VACCINATION AND PREVENTION: PROTECTING YOUR LIVER FROM FURTHER DAMAGE

8.1 IMPORTANCE OF IMMUNIZATION: PROTECTING YOURSELF FROM VIRAL HEPATITIS

Your liver is a tireless defender, working around the clock to filter toxins and protect you from illness. However, some enemies, like viral hepatitis, require an extra layer of defense. This chapter will explore the importance of immunization for safeguarding yourself from various forms of viral hepatitis, empowering you to take charge of your liver health.

Understanding the Threat: A Closer Look at Viral Hepatitis

Viral hepatitis is a liver infection caused by different viruses. These viruses can damage liver cells, leading to inflammation, scarring (cirrhosis), and even liver failure in severe cases. Here's a breakdown of the most common types of viral hepatitis:

1. Hepatitis A: This highly contagious virus typically spreads through contaminated food or water. While most people recover fully from hepatitis A, it can cause severe illness in some cases.

2. Hepatitis B: This virus spreads through bodily fluids like blood or semen. Chronic hepatitis B infection can lead to serious liver damage over time.

3. Hepatitis C: This bloodborne virus can also spread through sharing needles or other contaminated equipment. Chronic hepatitis C infection is a leading cause of liver cancer.

The Power of Prevention: Vaccines as Your Liver's Shield

Fortunately, vaccines are available to protect you from hepatitis A and B, significantly reducing your risk of infection. Here's how these vaccines work:

Exposing Your Body's Defenses: Vaccines contain a weakened or inactive form of the virus. When you receive a vaccination, your immune system recognizes this weakened virus and creates antibodies to fight it. This way, if you encounter the real virus in the future, your body is already prepared to attack it effectively.

Long-Term Protection: Hepatitis A and B vaccines offer long-lasting immunity, significantly reducing your risk of getting infected and developing serious liver complications.

Vaccination Recommendations: Who Should Get Vaccinated?

The Centers for Disease Control and Prevention (CDC) recommends the following:

Hepatitis A Vaccine: Everyone, regardless of age, should receive the hepatitis A vaccine. It's typically administered in two doses, with the second dose given six months to a year after the first.

Hepatitis B Vaccine: The hepatitis B vaccine is recommended for all infants, children, and adolescents. It's also recommended for adults at increased risk of infection, such as healthcare workers, travelers to certain regions, and people with multiple sexual partners.

Beyond the Basics: Additional Considerations

While the hepatitis A and B vaccines offer robust protection, here are some additional points to consider:

Hepatitis C Vaccine: Unfortunately, there is currently no vaccine available for hepatitis C. However, effective treatments can manage the infection and significantly reduce the risk of complications.

Booster Shots: For optimal protection against hepatitis B, booster shots may be recommended in certain cases. Consult your doctor to determine if you need a booster shot.

Talk to Your Doctor: If you have any questions or concerns about hepatitis vaccination, discuss them with your doctor. They can provide personalized guidance based on your age, health history, and risk factors.

Vaccination is one of the most effective ways to protect yourself and your loved ones from viral hepatitis. By getting vaccinated, you're giving your liver a powerful shield against these potentially harmful viruses, promoting optimal liver health and overall well-being.

8.2 Avoiding Toxins: Minimizing Exposure to Environmental Hazards

Your liver acts as your body's filtration system, working tirelessly to process nutrients, eliminate waste products, and neutralize toxins. However, in today's world, we're constantly exposed to environmental hazards that can overburden this vital organ. This chapter will explore ways to minimize your exposure to toxins and empower you to become an advocate for your liver health.

The Invisible Threat: Understanding Environmental Toxins

Environmental toxins encompass a wide range of chemicals and pollutants found in air, water, food, and consumer products. These toxins can enter your body through inhalation, ingestion, or skin absorption. Here are some common examples:

Air Pollutants: Traffic fumes, industrial emissions, and cigarette smoke contain harmful toxins that can damage your liver.

Contaminated Water: Drinking water can sometimes be contaminated with pesticides, industrial waste, or heavy metals, putting a strain on your liver's detoxification abilities.

Food Additives and Preservatives: Processed foods often contain artificial ingredients, preservatives, and unhealthy fats that can contribute to liver stress.

Household Toxins: Cleaning products, pesticides, and personal care products can harbor harmful chemicals that can be absorbed through the skin or inhaled.

The Domino Effect: How Toxins Impact Your Liver Health

Chronic exposure to environmental toxins can take a toll on your liver function in several ways:

Increased Workload: Your liver is constantly working to break down and eliminate toxins. Excessive exposure can overload your liver, hindering its ability to perform other essential functions.

Oxidative Stress: Many toxins generate free radicals, unstable molecules that damage your cells and contribute to inflammation. This oxidative stress can harm liver cells and promote fatty liver disease.

Hormonal Disruption: Certain environmental toxins can mimic or interfere with hormones, potentially leading to metabolic imbalances that can affect your liver health.

Empowering Yourself: Strategies for Minimizing Toxin Exposure

While we can't entirely eliminate exposure to environmental toxins, there are steps you can take to minimize your risk:

Improve Air Quality: Reduce indoor air pollution by using air purifiers and increasing ventilation. Limit exposure to secondhand smoke and avoid spending extended periods outdoors when air quality is poor.

Drink Clean Water: Invest in a good quality water filter to remove potential contaminants from your drinking water. You can also choose bottled spring water from reputable brands.

Eat a Whole-Foods Diet: Focus on consuming fresh, whole foods like fruits, vegetables, and whole grains. These foods are naturally low in toxins and rich in nutrients that support your liver's detoxification process.

Read Food Labels: Be mindful of ingredients when purchasing packaged foods. Limit intake of processed foods with artificial additives, preservatives, and unhealthy fats.

Choose Natural Cleaning Products: opt for eco-friendly cleaning products that are free of harsh chemicals. Look for natural alternatives like vinegar, baking soda, and lemon juice for everyday cleaning tasks.

Reduce Chemical Exposure in Personal Care Products: Many personal care products contain potentially harmful ingredients. Choose natural or organic alternatives whenever possible.

Support Toxin-Free Living: Advocate for stricter regulations on environmental pollutants and support companies committed to sustainable practices.

Small changes can make a big difference. By incorporating these strategies into your daily routine, you can significantly reduce your exposure to environmental toxins and empower your liver to function optimally.

8.3 Alcohol and Drugs: Understanding Their Impact on the Liver

Your liver is a resilient organ, but it has limits. This chapter will explore the impact of alcohol and drugs on your liver function, empowering you to make informed choices that protect this vital organ.

The Liver's Role in Processing Alcohol and Drugs

Think of your liver as a tireless detox center. When you consume alcohol or drugs, your liver goes into overdrive to break them down and remove them from your body. Here's a closer look at this process:

Alcohol Breakdown: The liver prioritizes processing alcohol. It breaks down alcohol into harmless byproducts, which are then eliminated from your body through urine or sweat.

Drug Detoxification: The liver also metabolizes many drugs, converting them into inactive forms that can be safely excreted.

The Downside of Overconsumption: How Excessive Alcohol and Drugs Harm Your Liver

While your liver can handle occasional indulgence, chronic or excessive consumption of alcohol and drugs can take a significant toll. Here's how:

Overworked and Overwhelmed: Excessive alcohol and drugs overload your liver, hindering its ability to perform other essential functions like processing nutrients and synthesizing proteins.

Toxic Byproducts: The breakdown of alcohol and some drugs can generate harmful byproducts. These byproducts can damage liver cells and trigger inflammation.

Fatty Liver Disease: Chronic alcohol and drug use can lead to the accumulation of fat in the liver, a condition known as fatty liver disease. Left untreated, fatty liver disease can progress to more serious conditions like cirrhosis and liver failure.

Scarring and Cirrhosis: Persistent damage from alcohol and drugs can cause scar tissue to form in the liver. Over time, this scar tissue can replace healthy liver tissue, leading to cirrhosis, a condition that significantly impairs liver function.

Understanding the Risks: Different Drugs and Their Impact

Not all drugs affect your liver equally. Here's a breakdown of some common categories and their potential risks:

Over-the-Counter Medications: While generally safe when used as directed, certain over-the-counter pain relievers and medications can damage your liver with high doses or prolonged use.

Prescription Medications: Some prescription medications can be hepatotoxic, meaning they can harm your liver. Always follow your doctor's instructions and discuss any potential liver risks associated with your medications.

Illegal Drugs: Illicit drugs like cocaine, heroin, and certain steroids can be particularly damaging to your liver.

Making Informed Choices for a Healthy Liver

The good news is that you have the power to protect your liver. Here are some strategies to consider:

Moderate Alcohol Consumption: If you choose to drink alcohol, do so in moderation. For most healthy adults, this means no more than one drink per day for women and two drinks per day for men.

Talk to Your Doctor About Medications: Discuss any medications you take, including over-the-counter and prescription drugs, with your doctor. They can advise you on potential liver risks and offer alternatives if necessary.

Avoid Illicit Drugs: Using illegal drugs is not only risky for your overall health but also poses a significant threat to your liver function.

Prioritize a Healthy Lifestyle: Maintaining a healthy weight, eating a balanced diet, and getting regular exercise all contribute to overall health and support your liver's ability to process substances.

Your liver is a remarkable organ, but it's not invincible. Being mindful of your alcohol and drug consumption and making informed choices can significantly reduce your risk of liver damage and promote long-term liver health.

CHAPTER NINE

MEDICATION MANAGEMENT: WORKING WITH YOUR DOCTOR

9.1 UNDERSTANDING YOUR MEDICATION REGIMEN: ADHERENCE AND POTENTIAL SIDE EFFECTS

Taking medications can be a crucial part of managing various health conditions. However, medications can sometimes have unintended consequences, especially for your liver, the body's primary detoxification organ. This chapter will empower you to understand your medication regimen, promote adherence, and navigate potential side effects for optimal liver health.

Working in Tandem: Medications and Your Liver

Many medications rely on your liver to break them down and eliminate them from your body. While medications are designed to improve your health, they can sometimes place additional stress on your liver. Here's a breakdown of the process:

The Liver's Detoxification Role: Your liver acts as a filter, processing nutrients, removing waste products, and breaking down foreign substances like medications.

Medication Metabolism: The liver converts medications into inactive forms that can be safely excreted through urine or stool. This process allows the medication to take effect and then be eliminated from the body.

The Importance of Adherence: Taking Your Medications as Prescribed

Following your doctor's instructions for taking your medications is crucial for both your overall health and liver function. Here's why adherence matters:

Effective Treatment: Taking your medications as prescribed ensures you receive the full therapeutic benefit. Skipping doses or not completing the entire course can render the medication ineffective.

Minimizing Side Effects: Taking medications as directed can help minimize potential side effects, including those that may impact your liver.

Protecting Your Liver: Following your medication regimen can prevent complications from your underlying health condition, which may ultimately protect your liver health.

Understanding Potential Side Effects: Working with Your Doctor

All medications can have side effects, some of which may affect your liver. Here's how to navigate potential side effects:

Review Medication Information: Carefully read the medication information leaflet that comes with your prescription. This leaflet will list potential side effects, including those related to the liver.

Communicate with Your Doctor: Discuss any side affects you experience with your doctor, even if they seem mild.

They can adjust your medication or recommend alternative treatments if necessary.

Be Proactive: Don't hesitate to ask your doctor questions about your medications and potential liver risks. The more informed you are, the better equipped you are to manage your health.

Strategies for Adherence: Developing a Medication Routine that Works for You

Taking medications consistently can be challenging, especially if you're juggling multiple prescriptions. Here are some strategies to promote adherence:

Set Reminders: Use alarms on your phone, pill organizers, or calendar reminders to help you remember to take your medications on time.

Develop a Routine: Incorporate medication into your daily routine, such as taking them at mealtimes or before bed. This can help you establish a consistent habit.

Simplify Your Regimen: Talk to your doctor about simplifying your medication regimen if possible. This could involve combining medications or switching to a long-acting medication that requires less frequent dosing.

Invest in a Pill Organizer: A pill organizer can help you keep track of your medications and ensure you have the correct dosage for each day.

Talk to Your Pharmacist: Your pharmacist can answer questions about your medications and offer tips for adhering to your regimen.

Remember: Communication is key. By working openly with your doctor and pharmacist, you can develop a medication plan that is safe, effective, and promotes optimal liver health. The next chapter will explore the world of food and delve into the best dietary practices to support your liver function. You'll learn about specific liver-friendly foods and strategies for creating a healthy and delicious eating plan.

9.2 Communicating Effectively: Discussing Concerns and Treatment Options with Your Doctor

Your doctor is your partner in health. When it comes to your liver health, open and effective communication is crucial. This chapter equips you with the tools to confidently discuss your concerns, navigate treatment options, and become an active participant in your healthcare journey.

The Power of Open Communication: Why Talking to Your Doctor Matters

Whether you're concerned about potential liver problems, managing an existing condition, or simply seeking guidance for optimal liver health, a productive conversation with your doctor is essential. Here's why open communication matters:

Accurate Diagnosis and Treatment: By sharing your symptoms, medical history, and lifestyle habits, you empower your doctor to make an accurate diagnosis and recommend the most appropriate treatment plan for your individual needs.

Addressing Your Concerns: Don't hesitate to voice any concerns you have about your liver health, medications, or potential side effects. Your doctor can address your worries and provide reassurance or explore alternative approaches if needed.

Informed Decision-Making: Open communication allows you to understand your treatment options and their potential benefits and risks. This empowers you to participate actively in decisions about your healthcare.

Building Trust and Collaboration: A trusting relationship with your doctor is vital for long-term health management. Effective communication fosters collaboration, allowing you to work together towards your health goals.

Effective Communication Strategies: From Preparation to Follow-Up

Here are some tips to ensure your conversations with your doctor regarding liver health are productive and informative:

- Preparation is Key: Before your appointment, write down your questions and concerns. List any medications you're taking, including over-the-counter drugs and supplements. Prepare a brief timeline of any symptoms you've been experiencing.

- Be Clear and Concise: Clearly state your concerns and questions. Use simple language and avoid medical jargon.

- Actively Listen: Pay close attention to your doctor's explanations and ask clarifying questions if needed. Take notes during the appointment if it helps you remember key information.

- Don't Be Afraid to Ask "Why": Understanding the rationale behind your treatment plan can empower you to feel more confident about your healthcare decisions.

- Express Your Preferences: If you have any preferences regarding treatment options, discuss them with your doctor. They can explain the pros and cons of each approach to help you make an informed decision.

- Follow Up: If you have any questions or concerns after your appointment, don't hesitate to follow up with your doctor's office.

Beyond Words: Nonverbal Communication also Matters

While verbal communication is essential, nonverbal cues also play a role in effective communication. Here are some tips to consider:

Maintain Eye Contact: Eye contact demonstrates attentiveness and respect.

Body Language: Open and relaxed body language signifies that you're engaged in the conversation.

Be Assertive, Not Aggressive: Clearly express your concerns, but maintain a respectful tone.

Remember: You are an advocate for your own health. By taking charge of communication with your doctor, you become a partner in your healthcare journey and ensure that your liver health receives the optimal level of attention and care.

9.3 Medication Management Tools: Strategies for Staying on Track

Juggling medications, especially those for chronic conditions, can feel overwhelming at times. This chapter equips you with practical tools and strategies to manage your medication regimen effectively, promoting optimal liver health and overall well-being.

The Importance of Medication Adherence for Liver Health

As discussed in previous chapters, medications can sometimes place additional stress on your liver as it processes and eliminates them. However, following your doctor's instructions for taking medications is crucial for both your overall health and liver function. Taking medications as prescribed ensures:

Effective Treatment: Skipping doses or not completing the full course can render the medication ineffective, potentially leading to complications that could further burden your liver.

Minimizing Side Effects: Following your medication regimen can help minimize potential side effects, including those that may impact your liver.

Protecting Your Liver: Taking medications as directed can help prevent complications from your underlying health condition, ultimately protecting your liver health.

Conquering the Chaos: Tools and Strategies for Effective Medication Management

Here are some practical tools and strategies to help you stay on track with your medication regimen:

Utilize Medication Reminders: Technology is your friend! Set alarms on your phone, download medication reminder apps, or invest in a talking pill dispenser. Visual cues like pill boxes with compartments for each day of the week can also be helpful.

Develop a Routine: Integrate medication into your daily routine. For example, take medications at mealtimes or before bed. This consistency makes it easier to form a habit.

Simplify Your Regimen: Talk to your doctor about simplifying your medication regimen if possible. This could involve combining medications or switching to long-acting versions that require less frequent dosing.

Involve Your Family or Caregivers: If you need help managing your medications, enlist the support of a family member or caregiver. They can help you set reminders or ensure you have the correct medications on hand.

Maintain a Medication List: Keep a comprehensive list of all your medications, including their names, dosages, and frequencies. Update this list regularly and share it with your doctor and pharmacist.

Track Your Progress: Consider using a medication tracker app or a simple paper log to document when you take your medications. This can help you identify any missed doses and ensure you're staying on schedule.

Prepare for Travel: When traveling, plan ahead. Pack an extra supply of your medications and keep them in your carry-on luggage in case of checked baggage delays.

Obtain a doctor's note for any medications you need to bring on the plane.

Address Medication Concerns: Don't hesitate to talk to your doctor or pharmacist if you have any questions or concerns about your medications, such as potential side effects or interactions with other substances.

Beyond the Tools: Building Sustainable Habits for Long-Term Success

Medication adherence is a marathon, not a sprint. Here are some additional tips for building sustainable habits and staying on track with your medications long-term:

Focus on the Benefits: Remind yourself of the positive reasons you're taking your medications. They are helping you manage your health and improve your overall well-being.

Reward Yourself: Small rewards can be motivating. Celebrate your adherence milestones with a healthy treat or an activity you enjoy.

Find a Support System: Talk to friends, family, or a support group about your challenges with medication adherence. Sharing your experiences can be motivating and help you feel less alone.

Address Underlying Issues: Sometimes, forgetfulness or difficulty sticking to a routine can stem from other factors like stress or depression. If you suspect an underlying issue, talk to your doctor for additional support.

Effective medication management is a skill that takes time and practice to master. Be patient with yourself, celebrate your successes, and don't be afraid to seek help if you need it. By staying on track with your medications, you're taking an important step towards optimal liver health and a healthier you.

CHAPTER TEN

BUILDING A HAPPY LIFE

10.1 THE POWER OF CONNECTION: JOINING SUPPORT GROUPS AND ONLINE COMMUNITIES

Living with a health condition, especially one that affects a vital organ like your liver, can feel isolating at times. This chapter explores the power of connection and the benefits of joining support groups and online communities dedicated to liver health.

The Human Connection: Why Support Matters

Whether you're newly diagnosed with a liver condition or managing a chronic condition, navigating the complexities of healthcare and lifestyle changes can be overwhelming. Support groups and online communities offer a safe space to connect with others who understand your journey. Here's why connection matters:

Shared Experiences: Connecting with others who have similar experiences can be incredibly validating. You'll realize you're not alone and gain a sense of community.

Emotional Support: Support groups and online communities offer a platform to share your concerns, frustrations, and triumphs. The understanding and encouragement you receive can be a source of strength.

Information Exchange: These groups can be valuable sources of information about liver health, treatment options, and coping strategies. Members can share their experiences with different medications, specialists, and alternative therapies.

Motivation and Inspiration: Seeing others successfully manage their liver health can be incredibly motivating. You can learn from their experiences and gain inspiration to stay on track with your own health goals.

Finding the Right Fit: Exploring Different Types of Support

There are various ways to connect with others who share your interest in liver health. Here's a breakdown of some options:

In-Person Support Groups: Local hospitals, community centers, and patient advocacy organizations often host in-person support groups. These groups allow for face-to-face interaction and can foster a strong sense of community.

Online Support Groups: Several online platforms host liver health support groups. These groups offer the convenience of participating from the comfort of your own home and connecting with people from all over the world.

Social Media Groups: Many social media platforms have dedicated groups focused on liver health. These groups can be a source of information, support, and inspiration.

Building Connections: Tips for Participating in Support Groups and Online Communities

Whether you choose in-person or online support, here are some tips for maximizing your experience:

Do Your Research: Look for groups specific to your liver condition or area of interest. Some groups may be geared towards specific demographics, such as young adults or those with a particular diagnosis.

Start by Listening: Take some time to observe the group dynamic and listen to the experiences of others before actively participating.

Be Respectful and Open-Minded: Everyone's journey is unique. Respect different perspectives and experiences within the group.

Share Your Story When You're Ready: Don't feel pressured to share personal information immediately. Participate at your own pace and comfort level.

Focus on Positive Interactions: While it's important to acknowledge challenges, focus on finding support and encouragement within the group.

Seek Professional Help if Needed: Support groups and online communities are not a substitute for professional medical advice. If you have any questions or concerns, consult your doctor.

Beyond Support: The Power of Advocacy

Many online communities and support groups also champion liver health awareness and advocacy. You can get involved in:

Raising Awareness: Sharing your story or participating in advocacy campaigns can help raise awareness about liver health and the importance of early diagnosis.

Supporting Research: Some organizations connected to support groups raise funds for liver health research. You can contribute financially or volunteer your time to support these efforts.

Connection is a powerful tool on your journey towards optimal liver health. By joining a support group or online community, you gain access to valuable information, emotional support, and a sense of belonging. You'll discover that you're not alone, and together, you can navigate your health journey with greater confidence and strength.

10.2 Talking to Loved Ones: Open Communication and Emotional Support

Your liver health is intricately linked to your overall well-being. Beyond medical interventions and lifestyle choices, the support of loved ones plays a crucial role in navigating health challenges. This chapter explores the importance of open communication with your family and friends and how their understanding and encouragement can empower you on your journey towards optimal liver health.

Building Bridges of Understanding: Why Talking to Loved Ones Matters

Whether you're newly diagnosed with a liver condition or managing a chronic condition, talking to your loved ones about your health can be empowering. Here's why open communication matters:

Reduced Stress and Anxiety: Sharing your concerns and challenges with loved ones can alleviate feelings of isolation and provide a sense of emotional release. Talking things through can help you manage stress and anxiety, which can have a positive impact on your overall health.

Increased Support: By openly discussing your needs, you empower your loved ones to offer practical and emotional support. This could involve assistance with healthy meal preparation, transportation to appointments, or simply a listening ear.

Improved Treatment Adherence: Talking to your loved ones about your medications and treatment plan can help them hold you accountable and celebrate your successes. Their encouragement can be a powerful motivator to stay on track with your health goals.

Building a Support System: Living with a health condition can be challenging. Open communication fosters a sense of shared responsibility and creates a support system you can rely on during difficult times.

Communication Strategies: Sharing Your Story with Empathy and Clarity

Talking about your health can feel daunting. Here are some strategies to facilitate open communication with your loved ones:

Choose the Right Time and Place: Find a private, relaxed setting where you can have a conversation without distractions.

Start by Sharing Your Feelings: Express your emotions honestly, whether it's fear, frustration, or uncertainty.

Provide Information: Educate your loved ones about your liver condition, treatment plan, and any dietary restrictions you may have. Use clear and concise language, avoiding medical jargon if possible. Offer resources like websites or articles they can explore for further information.

Focus on Your Needs: Clearly communicate the kind of support you need, whether it's practical help with tasks or simply a listening ear.

Be Patient with Understanding: It may take time for your loved ones to fully grasp your situation. Be patient and answer their questions honestly.

Focus on the Positive: While acknowledging challenges, emphasize your hope for the future and your commitment to managing your health.

Fostering a Supportive Environment: Tips for Loved Ones

If you have a loved one living with a liver condition, here are some ways you can offer support:

Listen Actively: Pay attention to their concerns and feelings without judgment. Offer empathy and a safe space for them to express themselves.

Educate Yourself: Learn more about their condition and its treatments. This knowledge will help you understand their challenges and provide more informed support.

Offer Practical Help: Assist with tasks like grocery shopping, preparing healthy meals, or driving them to appointments. Small acts of kindness can make a big difference.

Respect Their Boundaries: Be mindful of their energy levels and respect their need for privacy. Don't be pushy or try to force them to talk when they're not ready.

Celebrate Their Victories: Acknowledge their efforts to manage their health, no matter how small. Positive reinforcement can be a powerful motivator.

Maintain a Positive Attitude: Your optimism and encouragement can be a source of strength for your loved one.

Open communication and emotional support from loved ones are vital for navigating any health challenge, including those affecting your liver. By talking openly and honestly, and by offering and accepting support with empathy and understanding, you can create a strong support system that empowers you to manage your health and live a fulfilling life.

10.3 Finding Inspiration: Stories of Resilience and Living Well

Living with a liver condition can feel isolating at times. This chapter aims to inspire you by sharing stories of resilience and the power of a positive attitude. You'll encounter individuals who have navigated their health challenges and found ways to live fulfilling lives. Their stories are a testament to the human spirit's ability to overcome adversity and a reminder that you are not alone on your journey towards optimal liver health.

Strength in Numbers: The Value of Shared Experiences

Reading about the experiences of others who have faced similar challenges can be incredibly motivating. These stories offer a glimpse into the realities of living with a liver condition, but also highlight the power of resilience, adaptation, and the importance of a positive outlook.

Angela's Story: Diagnosed with autoimmune hepatitis as a young adult, Angela faced years of uncertainty and treatment adjustments. However, she focused on building a strong support network, embraced a healthy lifestyle, and even started a blog to share her experiences and connect with others living with chronic liver conditions. Today, Angela leads an active life and advocates for increased awareness about liver health.

Michael's Journey: After receiving a liver transplant due to end-stage liver disease, Michael faced a long recovery process and the challenges of lifelong medication. He credits his positive attitude, his dedication to healthy habits, and the unwavering support of his family with helping him overcome adversity. Michael now volunteers with transplant support groups, inspiring others facing similar journeys.

David's Transformation: David struggled with fatty liver disease for years, fueled by unhealthy eating habits and a sedentary lifestyle. However, a wake-up call from his doctor prompted a significant change. David embraced a whole-foods diet, started exercising regularly, and found a renewed passion for life. He now inspires others to take control of their health and prioritize liver-friendly choices.

Finding Inspiration in Everyday Life

Inspiration doesn't have to come from grand gestures. Sometimes, the most inspiring stories are those of everyday individuals making small, consistent changes for the better:

The Determined Chef: Imagine a chef who, after being diagnosed with a liver condition, completely revamped their restaurant menu to focus on healthy, liver-friendly dishes, proving that delicious food can also be good for your liver.

The Active Gardener: Picture a retiree who, despite limitations due to a chronic liver condition, cultivates a beautiful vegetable garden, ensuring access to fresh, nutritious produce and a sense of accomplishment.

The Artful Yogi: Think of someone who uses gentle yoga practices to manage stress and improve overall well-being, showcasing the mind-body connection and its positive impact on liver health.

Remember: Every individual's journey is unique. These stories are meant to offer encouragement and hope. Focus on the aspects that resonate with you and find inspiration in the small victories and positive choices that others have made to improve their liver health and overall well-being.

The Power Within You: Taking Charge of Your Health

The stories in this chapter highlight the importance of:

Maintaining a Positive Attitude: A positive outlook can significantly impact your well-being and your ability to cope with challenges.

Building a Support System: Surrounding yourself with supportive loved ones can provide emotional strength and practical assistance.

Embracing Healthy Habits: Prioritizing a nutritious diet, regular exercise, and stress management practices are crucial for optimal liver health.

Taking Control: Educate yourself about your condition, advocate for your needs, and become an active participant in your healthcare journey.

You are not defined by your liver condition. You have the power to make choices that support your health and well-being. By taking inspiration from others and focusing on your own strengths, you can navigate your journey towards optimal liver health with resilience, optimism, and a renewed sense of purpose.

CHAPTER ELEVEN

LIVING YOUR BEST LIFE WITH LIVER DISEASE

11.1 MAKING ADJUSTMENTS: ADAPTING ACTIVITIES AND TRAVEL CONSIDERATIONS

Living with a liver condition doesn't mean giving up on your passions and interests. This chapter explores strategies for adapting activities you enjoy and navigating travel while prioritizing optimal liver health.

Finding Balance: Adapting Activities, You Love

Many activities you enjoy can still be part of your life with a few adjustments. Here's how to strike a balance:

Listen to Your Body: Be mindful of your energy levels and limitations. Don't push yourself too hard, and take breaks when needed.

Focus on Quality Over Quantity: Modify activities to fit your current capabilities. For example, if you love hiking, choose shorter, less strenuous trails.

Explore New Activities: Consider activities that are gentler on your body, such as yoga, swimming, or tai chi. You might discover new passions that complement your overall well-being.

Communicate and Collaborate: Talk to friends and family about adapting activities you do together. They may be willing to adjust plans to accommodate your needs.

Finding Common Ground: Considerations for Safe and Enjoyable Travel

Traveling can be an enriching experience, but it's important to prioritize your liver health when planning a trip. Here are some key considerations:

Consult Your Doctor: Before booking your trip, discuss your travel plans with your doctor. They can advise on potential risks and necessary precautions, and ensure your medications are refilled for the duration of your trip.

Choose Your Destination Wisely: Consider factors like climate, access to clean water and healthy food options, and availability of medical care when selecting your travel destination.

Pack Smart: Pack a sufficient supply of medications and any necessary medical supplies, like syringes or glucose tablets if you have diabetes. Bring a doctor's note explaining your condition and medications in case you encounter any issues at customs.

Plan for Rest and Relaxation: Factor in plenty of rest and relaxation time during your travels. Avoid overexerting yourself and prioritize activities that are manageable for your energy levels.

Be Mindful of Food and Beverages: Research food safety standards at your destination and stick to bottled or boiled water. Choose familiar, healthy foods to minimize the risk of digestive issues. Be moderate with alcohol consumption and avoid unhygienic street food.

Maintain Healthy Habits: As much as possible, stick to your regular healthy habits while traveling. Pack healthy snacks, stay hydrated, and prioritize sleep.

Remember: Communication is key. Talk openly with travel agents, tour operators, and accommodation providers about your needs. Many travel companies offer options for health-conscious travelers or those with specific dietary requirements.

Making Adjustments, Not Sacrifices

Adapting activities and travel plans doesn't have to feel like a sacrifice. By approaching these situations creatively and with open communication, you can still enjoy the activities you love and explore the world while prioritizing your liver health. The next chapter dives into the delicious world of food and explores the best dietary practices to support your liver function. You'll learn about specific liver-friendly foods and strategies for creating a healthy and enjoyable eating plan.

11.2 Finding Joy and Purpose: Maintaining a Positive Outlook and Embracing Life

Living with a liver condition can present challenges, but it doesn't have to define your life. This chapter focuses on cultivating a positive outlook and embracing life's possibilities. By nurturing your well-being and fostering a sense of purpose, you can navigate your health journey with greater resilience and joy.

The Power of Positivity: Why a Positive Attitude Matters

A positive outlook isn't just about feeling good. Studies have shown that optimism can have a significant impact on your physical and mental health. Here's why a positive attitude matter:

Stress Management: Positive thinking can help you manage stress more effectively, which can benefit your overall health and well-being, including your liver function.

Improved Treatment Outcomes: A positive attitude can influence your treatment journey. People with a more optimistic outlook are often more likely to adhere to treatment plans and experience better overall health outcomes.

Enhanced Quality of Life: Focusing on the positive aspects of life can increase your happiness and enjoyment of daily activities.

Cultivating Optimism: Practical Strategies for a Positive Mindset

Developing a positive outlook is a journey, not a destination. Here are some practical strategies to cultivate optimism:

Practice Gratitude: Take time each day to appreciate the good things in your life, no matter how small. Keeping a gratitude journal can be a helpful tool.

Focus on What You Can Control: Focus your energy on the aspects of your life that you can control, such as your diet, exercise routine, and stress management practices. Let go of things outside your control.

Challenge Negative Thoughts: When negative thoughts arise, challenge their validity. Replace them with more positive and realistic self-talk.

Surround Yourself with Positivity: Spend time with supportive and optimistic people who uplift and inspire you.

Find Humor in Everyday Life: Laughter is a powerful stress reliever and can boost your mood. Find humor in everyday situations and enjoy lighthearted moments.

Practice Mindfulness: Mindfulness practices like meditation or deep breathing can help you stay present in the moment and appreciate the simple joys of life.

Living with Purpose: Finding Meaning and Fulfillment

Having a sense of purpose goes beyond simply existing. It's about feeling connected to something bigger than yourself and finding fulfillment in your life. Here's how to explore your purpose:

Reflect on Your Values: Consider what matters most to you in life. Is it creativity, helping others, learning new things, or spending time with loved ones? Identifying your core values can guide you towards activities that bring you meaning.

Explore Your Passions: What are you naturally drawn to? Do you enjoy writing, playing music, volunteering, or spending time in nature? Engage in activities that spark your joy and ignite your passions.

Set Goals and Challenges: Setting achievable goals can give you a sense of direction and accomplishment. These goals can be related to your health, hobbies, relationships, or personal growth.

Help Others: Helping others is a proven way to boost happiness and fulfillment. Volunteer your time, mentor someone, or simply perform acts of kindness in your everyday life.

Embrace Lifelong Learning: Never stop learning and growing. Take classes, read books, or explore new hobbies. Learning new things keeps your mind sharp and opens doors to new possibilities.

cultivating a positive outlook and embracing a sense of purpose, you can find joy, meaning, and fulfillment in your life, even with health challenges. The next chapter dives into the delicious world of food and explores the best dietary practices to support your liver function. You'll learn about specific liver-friendly foods and strategies for creating a healthy and enjoyable eating plan.

11.3 Setting Realistic Goals: Achieving What Matters Most Despite Challenges

Living with a liver condition can sometimes feel overwhelming. This chapter empowers you to take control by setting realistic and achievable goals for optimal liver health. By establishing clear objectives and focusing on progress over perfection, you can navigate your health journey with a sense of accomplishment and motivation.

The Power of Goal Setting: Why It Matters

Setting goals is a powerful tool for positive change. Here's how clearly defined goals can benefit your journey towards optimal liver health:

Increased Motivation: Having specific goals provides direction and keeps you motivated to make healthy choices.

Improved Focus: Goals help you prioritize actions that contribute to your overall health and well-being.

Enhanced Self-Confidence: Achieving goals, big or small, builds self-confidence and a sense of accomplishment.

Progress Tracking: Goals provide a framework for measuring progress and celebrating your victories, no matter how small.

The Art of SMART Goals: Setting Yourself Up for Success

Not all goals are created equal. When setting goals for liver health, it's important to follow the SMART criteria:

Specific: Clearly define your goals. Instead of a vague goal like "eat healthier," aim for "eat at least three servings of vegetables per day."

Measurable: Establish a way to track your progress. This could involve logging your food intake, recording exercise sessions, or using a weight-loss app.

Attainable: Set goals that are challenging but achievable. Don't overwhelm yourself with unrealistic expectations.

Relevant: Ensure your goals align with your overall health objectives and doctor's recommendations.

Time-Bound: Set a timeframe for achieving your goals. This creates a sense of urgency and helps you stay on track.

Breaking Down Big Goals into Smaller Steps

Large, daunting goals can feel paralyzing. Here's how to make them more manageable:

Chunk It Down: Break down your long-term goals into smaller, more achievable milestones. Celebrate reaching each milestone to stay motivated.

Focus on Habits: Long-term success hinges on establishing healthy habits. Focus on building small, sustainable changes into your daily routine.

Prioritize Progress: Don't get discouraged by setbacks. Focus on progress, not perfection. Even small improvements contribute to your overall health.

Examples of SMART Goals for Liver Health

Here are some examples of SMART goals you can set for yourself:

Increase vegetable intake: "I will include at least two servings of vegetables in my lunch and dinner meals for the next two weeks."

Reduce sugary drinks: "I will replace sugary drinks with water or unsweetened tea for the next month."

Increase physical activity: "I will go for a 30-minute walk three times a week for the next three months."

Improve sleep hygiene: "I will establish a regular sleep schedule and aim for 7-8 hours of sleep per night for the next four weeks."

Learn about liver health: "I will read one article about liver-friendly foods each week for the next month."

Remember: Setting goals is a personal journey. Adapt these examples to fit your specific needs, preferences, and doctor's recommendations.

Building a Support System for Goal Achievement

Having a support system can make a world of difference in achieving your goals. Here's how to leverage your network:

Share Your Goals: Tell your loved ones, friends, or a support group about your goals. Their encouragement and understanding can be a powerful motivator.

Find an Accountability Partner: Consider partnering with a friend or family member who is also working on health goals. Hold each other accountable and celebrate successes together.

Seek Professional Support: Don't hesitate to seek help from a registered dietitian, nutritionist, or fitness professional for personalized guidance.

Setting realistic goals and taking consistent action are key to sustainable change. By focusing on progress, celebrating your victories, and seeking support when needed, you can empower yourself to achieve your optimal liver health goals. The next chapter dives into the delicious world of food and explores the best dietary practices to support your liver function. You'll learn about specific liver-friendly foods and strategies for creating a healthy and enjoyable eating plan.

CHAPTER TWELVE

LIVER HEALTH FOR THE FUTURE: ADVOCACY AND RESEARCH UPDATES

12.1 STAYING INFORMED: RESOURCES FOR LIVER HEALTH EDUCATION AND ADVOCACY

Living with a liver condition requires ongoing education and a proactive approach to managing your health. This chapter empowers you by providing valuable resources for liver health education and advocacy. By staying informed and getting involved, you can take control of your health journey and contribute to a better understanding of liver disease.

Building Your Knowledge Base: Trustworthy Resources for Learning

The internet offers a wealth of information, but it's crucial to rely on credible sources. Here are some trustworthy resources to get you started:

National Institutes of Health (NIH): The National Institutes of Health (NIH) provides a comprehensive website with information on various liver diseases, including causes, symptoms, diagnosis, and treatment options. They also offer resources on clinical trials and patient education materials: National Institutes of Health (NIH)

American Liver Foundation (ALF): The American Liver Foundation (ALF) is a leading national organization dedicated to promoting liver health and advocacy. Their website offers a wealth of information on various liver conditions, healthy living tips, and resources for patients and caregivers: American Liver Foundation (ALF)

American Association for the Study of Liver Diseases (AASLD): The American Association for the Study of Liver Diseases (AASLD) is a professional society focused on advancing research and education in liver disease. Their website provides access to the latest research findings and clinical practice guidelines: American Association for the Study of Liver Diseases (AASLD)

LiverMD: LiverMD is a patient education website created by a team of liver specialists. It offers in-depth information on a variety of liver conditions, presented in a clear and understandable way: LiverMD

Beyond Websites: Books, Support Groups, and Medical Professionals

In addition to online resources, consider exploring these avenues for learning:

Books and Articles: Numerous books and articles discuss liver health and specific liver conditions. Consult your doctor or librarian for recommendations on reputable sources.

Support Groups: Connecting with others living with liver conditions can be a valuable source of information and emotional support. Many support groups host educational sessions or have access to educational materials.

Doctor's Appointments: Your doctor is your primary source of information and guidance. Don't hesitate to ask questions and express any concerns you may have.

Information is power, but it's important to discuss any new information you find with your doctor to ensure it aligns with your individual treatment plan.

Becoming an Advocate: Raising Awareness and Supporting Change

Knowledge isn't just power, it's also an opportunity to make a difference. Here's how you can become an advocate for liver health:

Share Your Story: Raising awareness about liver disease can help break down stigmas and encourage others to seek help. Consider sharing your story with friends, family, or on a support group forum.

Support Advocacy Organizations: Several organizations advocate for increased research funding, improved access to treatment, and better public awareness of liver disease. Donate your time or resources to these organizations.

Contact Your Legislators: Let your elected officials know about the importance of liver health research and funding. You can find contact information for your representatives online.

Your voice matters. By advocating for change, you can help create a future where better treatments and a deeper understanding of liver disease exist.

The Power of Community: Finding Support and Connection

The journey toward optimal liver health doesn't have to be a solitary one. This chapter will explore the valuable role of support groups and online communities in providing encouragement, information, and a sense of belonging. The next chapter dives into the delicious world of food and explores the best dietary practices to support your liver function. You'll learn about specific liver-friendly foods and strategies for creating a healthy and enjoyable eating plan.

12.2 Clinical Trials: Understanding the Role of Research in Liver Disease Management

The world of medicine is constantly evolving, and research plays a vital role in advancing our understanding and treatment of liver disease. This chapter explores the concept of clinical trials and how your participation can contribute to breakthroughs in liver health.

On the Forefront of Discovery: What are Clinical Trials?

Clinical trials are research studies that evaluate the safety and effectiveness of new medications, treatment approaches, or medical devices. They are meticulously designed and conducted to ensure the safety and well-being of participants.

There are different phases of clinical trials:

1. Phase I: These initial trials involve a small group of healthy volunteers to assess the safety and basic properties of a new treatment.

2. Phase II: Phase II trials involve a larger group of people with the specific liver condition to evaluate the effectiveness of the treatment and identify any potential side effects.

3. Phase III: These larger-scale trials compare the new treatment to a standard treatment or placebo to determine its effectiveness and gather further data on safety and side effects.

4. Phase IV: These ongoing studies monitor the long-term effects and safety of a treatment once it's been approved for use by the general population.

Why Participate in a Clinical Trial?

There are many compelling reasons to consider participating in a clinical trial:

Contributing to Medical Progress: By volunteering for a clinical trial, you play a vital role in advancing research and potentially improving the lives of others with liver disease.

Access to Leading-Edge Treatments: Clinical trials often provide access to new medications or treatment approaches that may not yet be widely available.

Close Monitoring and Expert Care: Participants in clinical trials receive regular monitoring and care from healthcare professionals at the forefront of liver disease research.

Potential for Improvement: Clinical trials offer the chance to experience a treatment that may be more effective than the current standard of care.

Understanding the Considerations: Is a Clinical Trial Right for You?

Clinical trials aren't for everyone. Here are some factors to consider when making a decision:

Your Specific Condition: Not every clinical trial is relevant to every liver condition. Ensure the trial focuses on a condition you have or are at risk for.

Inclusion and Exclusion Criteria: Each trial has specific criteria for who can participate. These criteria may consider factors like age, medical history, and current medications.

Potential Risks and Side Effects: No treatment is without risks. Carefully review the potential side effects associated with the treatment being studied in the trial.

Time Commitment: Clinical trials often require regular visits to the research center, which can be time-consuming. Consider your schedule and ability to commit to the required follow-up appointments.

Finding a Clinical Trial: Matching Your Needs with Research Opportunities

If you're interested in participating in a clinical trial, here are some resources to get you started:

ClinicalTrials.gov: This is a U.S. government website that provides a searchable database of clinical trials across the country. You can filter your search by location, condition, and other criteria.

National Institutes of Health (NIH): The NIH website offers information about clinical trials specifically related to liver disease research.

Patient Advocacy Organizations: Many patient advocacy organizations for liver disease maintain lists of ongoing clinical trials relevant to their specific condition.

Your doctor: Discuss your interest in clinical trials with your doctor. They can help you determine if there are any ongoing trials that might be a good fit for you.

Participation in a clinical trial is a personal decision. Weigh the potential benefits and risks carefully, and don't hesitate to ask your doctor any questions you may have.

Empowering the Future: Your Role in Liver Disease Research

By participating in clinical trials, you become an active partner in shaping the future of liver health. Your contribution can pave the way for better treatments and improved outcomes for people living with liver disease. The next chapter dives into the delicious world of food and explores the best dietary practices to support your liver function. You'll learn about specific liver-friendly foods and strategies for creating a healthy and enjoyable eating plan.

12.3 Hope for the Future: New Developments and Emerging Therapies

The field of liver disease research is constantly evolving, with exciting new developments offering a beacon of hope for the future. This chapter explores some promising advancements and emerging therapies that hold the potential to revolutionize liver health.

On the Cusp of Transformation: Paving the Way for Improved Treatment Options

Here's a glimpse into some of the groundbreaking advancements in liver disease research:

Gene Therapy: Gene therapy offers the potential to treat liver diseases caused by genetic mutations. This approach involves introducing healthy genes into liver cells to correct the underlying genetic defect.

Immunotherapy: Immunotherapy harnesses the power of the body's immune system to fight liver disease. This approach is being explored for autoimmune liver diseases and viral hepatitis.

Cell-Based Therapies: Researchers are investigating the use of stem cells or other types of cells to regenerate damaged liver tissue. These holds promise for improving liver function and potentially reversing liver damage.

Novel Antiviral Medications: New classes of antiviral medications are being developed to combat chronic viral hepatitis infections like hepatitis B and C. These medications aim to achieve a functional cure, meaning the virus remains undetectable in the body without the need for lifelong treatment.

Non-Invasive Diagnostic Techniques: New non-invasive methods for diagnosing and monitoring liver disease are being developed. These techniques aim to provide more accurate and less invasive alternatives to traditional liver biopsies.

The Power of Precision Medicine: Tailoring Treatments to Individual Needs

The concept of precision medicine is transforming healthcare, and liver disease is no exception. This approach aims to personalize treatment plans based on individual genetic makeup and the specific characteristics of the disease. By understanding the unique molecular makeup of a patient's liver condition, doctors can tailor treatments for optimal effectiveness and minimize side effects.

The Future of Liver Transplantation: Minimally Invasive Techniques and Expanding Donor Options

Liver transplantation remains a life-saving option for patients with end-stage liver disease. However, advancements are being made to improve transplant outcomes and increase access to this life-saving procedure:

Minimally Invasive Techniques: Laparoscopic and robotic-assisted surgical techniques are being used for liver transplantation, resulting in faster recovery times and less pain for patients.

Expanding Donor Options: Researchers are exploring ways to expand the pool of available donor livers. This may involve using organs from deceased donors with fatty livers or utilizing techniques to preserve donor livers for longer periods.

Xenotransplantation: Xenotransplantation, the transplantation of organs from animals to humans, is a potential future option. Researchers are investigating the use of pig livers for transplantation, but significant hurdles remain before this becomes a reality.

While some of these advancements are still in the early stages of development, they offer a glimpse into the exciting future of liver disease treatment. These new therapies hold the promise of improved outcomes, better quality of life, and potentially even cures for various liver conditions.

Looking Forward with Optimism: Embracing the Power of Research

The ongoing research in liver disease is a testament to the tireless efforts of scientists, doctors, and patient advocates.

By staying informed about these advancements and considering participation in clinical trials, you can become an active participant in shaping a future where liver disease is effectively managed and potentially even eradicated. The next chapter delves into the delicious world of food and explores the best dietary practices to support your liver function. You'll learn about specific liver-friendly foods and strategies for creating a healthy and enjoyable eating plan.

CONCLUSION

Living with a liver condition can present challenges, but it doesn't have to define your life. Throughout this book, you've explored the intricate workings of your liver, delved into the complexities of various liver conditions, and discovered a wealth of resources to guide you on your health journey.

This path may not always be smooth, but remember, you are not alone. The knowledge you've gained empowers you to make informed decisions about your health. The stories of resilience and the power of a positive outlook serve as a constant source of inspiration.

As you embark on this journey of optimal liver health, embrace these key takeaways:

Become an active participant in your healthcare: Don't hesitate to ask questions, express concerns, and work collaboratively with your doctor to create a personalized treatment plan.

Prioritize a healthy lifestyle: Nourish your body with liver-friendly foods, stay active, and prioritize quality sleep. These choices contribute significantly to your overall well-being.

Build a strong support system: Surround yourself with loved ones who offer encouragement and understanding. Consider joining a support group to connect with others who share similar experiences.

Embrace a positive outlook: A positive mindset can significantly impact your physical and mental health. Practice gratitude, focus on what you can control, and find joy in the simple things.

Stay informed and engaged: Knowledge is power. Utilize credible resources to learn more about liver health, and consider participating in clinical trials to contribute to advancements in liver disease research.

Living well with a liver condition is a journey, not a destination. There will be ups and downs along the way, but by focusing on progress over perfection, celebrating your victories, and embracing a proactive approach, you can navigate this journey with resilience, optimism, and a renewed sense of empowerment.

Recall, your liver is a remarkable organ with an incredible capacity for regeneration. By taking care of yourself and prioritizing your health, you empower your liver to function optimally and live a long and fulfilling life.

This book has served as a guide, but your journey continues. Embrace the delicious world of liver-friendly foods, and embark on a culinary adventure that nourishes your body and delights your taste buds. Remember, healthy eating doesn't have to be bland or boring. With a little creativity and planning, you can create delicious meals that support your liver health and leave you feeling satisfied.

Good appetite and best wishes on your journey towards optimal liver health!

GLOSSARY

- Antiviral medication: Drugs used to combat viral infections, including hepatitis B and C.

- Ascites: Abnormal buildup of fluid in the abdomen, a potential complication of liver disease.

- Autoimmune hepatitis: A condition where the immune system attacks the liver.

- Biopsy: A procedure where a small sample of tissue is removed for examination.

- Cirrhosis: Scarring of the liver that hinders its function.

- Clinical trial: A research study that evaluates the safety and effectiveness of new treatments.

- Diet: The foods and drinks a person consume regularly.

- End-stage liver disease: Severe liver damage where the liver can no longer function effectively.

- Enzyme: A protein that speeds up chemical reactions in the body. (e.g., AST, ALT)

- Fatty liver disease: A buildup of fat in the liver cells.

- Fibrosis: Scarring of tissue.

- Gene therapy: A technique that aims to treat genetic diseases by introducing healthy genes into cells.

- Hepatitis: Inflammation of the liver, often caused by viruses.

- Hepatocellular carcinoma (HCC): The most common type of liver cancer.

- Immunotherapy: Treatment that harnesses the body's immune system to fight disease.

- Inflammation: The body's response to injury or infection, characterized by swelling, redness, and pain.

- Liver function test (LFT): A blood test that assesses how well the liver is functioning.

- Non-invasive: A medical procedure that doesn't involve breaking the skin.

- Nutrition: The process of taking in and utilizing food for growth and maintenance of the body.

- Optimal liver health: The state where the liver functions at its best capacity.

- Precision medicine: A personalized approach to treatment based on individual genetic makeup.

- Proactive: Taking action to anticipate and prevent problems.

- Regeneration: The ability of an organ or tissue to repair and replace damaged cells.

- Support group: A group of people who offer encouragement and share experiences related to a specific health condition.

- Transplantation: A surgical procedure where an organ or tissue is removed from one person (donor) and placed into another person (recipient).

- Ultrasound: An imaging technique that uses sound waves to create a picture of the inside of the body.

- Viral hepatitis: Liver inflammation caused by a virus.

"Thanks for reading! If you enjoyed this book or found it useful, I'd be very grateful if you'd post a short review on Amazon. Your support really does make a difference and I read all the reviews personally so I can get your feedback and make this book even better.

9 79832 69749 76